Feature Papers in Diabetology 2023

Feature Papers in Diabetology 2023

Editor

Peter Clifton

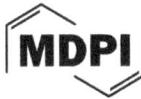

Basel • Beijing • Wuhan • Barcelona • Belgrade • Novi Sad • Cluj • Manchester

Editor
Peter Clifton
University of South Australia
Adelaide
Australia

Editorial Office
MDPI AG
Grosspeteranlage 5
4052 Basel, Switzerland

This is a reprint of articles from the Special Issue published online in the open access journal *Diabetology* (ISSN 2673-4540) (available at: https://www.mdpi.com/journal/diabetology/special_issues/8H78YJ5R54).

For citation purposes, cite each article independently as indicated on the article page online and as indicated below:

Lastname, A.A.; Lastname, B.B. Article Title. *Journal Name* **Year**, *Volume Number*, Page Range.

ISBN 978-3-7258-1939-3 (Hbk)
ISBN 978-3-7258-1940-9 (PDF)
doi.org/10.3390/books978-3-7258-1940-9

© 2024 by the authors. Articles in this book are Open Access and distributed under the Creative Commons Attribution (CC BY) license. The book as a whole is distributed by MDPI under the terms and conditions of the Creative Commons Attribution-NonCommercial-NoDerivs (CC BY-NC-ND) license.

Contents

Aliyanet Isamara Porcayo Ascencio, Evangelina Morales Carmona, Jesús Morán Farías, Dulce Stephanie Guzmán Medina, Rebeca Galindo Salas and Leobardo Sauque Reyna
Prevalence of Peripheral Arterial Disease and Principal Associated Risk Factors in Patients with Type 2 Diabetes Mellitus: The IDON-Peripheral Arterial Disease Study
Reprinted from: *Diabetology* 2024, 5, 15, doi:10.3390/diabetology5020015 1

Roberto Da Ros, Roberta Assaloni, Andrea Michelli, Barbara Brunato, Enrica Barro, Marco Meloni and Cesare Miranda
Burden of Infected Diabetic Foot Ulcers on Hospital Admissions and Costs in a Third-Level Center
Reprinted from: *Diabetology* 2024, 5, 11, doi:10.3390/diabetology5020011 17

Maria Antonietta Taras, Sara Cherchi, Ilaria Campesi, Valentina Margarita, Gavino Carboni, Paola Rappelli and Giancarlo Tonolo
Utility of Flash Glucose Monitoring to Determine Glucose Variation Induced by Different Doughs in Persons with Type 2 Diabetes
Reprinted from: *Diabetology* 2024, 5, 10, doi:10.3390/diabetology5010010 27

Sanja Klobučar, Andrej Belančić, Iva Bukša, Nikolina Morić and Dario Rahelić
Effectiveness of Oral versus Injectable Semaglutide in Adults with Type 2 Diabetes: Results from a Retrospective Observational Study in Croatia
Reprinted from: *Diabetology* 2024, 5, 5, doi:10.3390/diabetology5010005 39

Martina Matovinović, Andrej Belančić, Juraj Jug, Filip Mustač, Maja Sirovica, Mihovil Santini, et al.
Does the Efficacy of Semaglutide Treatment Differ between Low-Risk and High-Risk Subgroups of Patients with Type 2 Diabetes and Obesity Based on SCORE2, SCORE2-Diabetes, and ASCVD Calculations?
Reprinted from: *Diabetology* 2024, 5, 3, doi:10.3390/diabetology5010003 48

D'Artagnan M. Robinson, Dalia Regos-Stewart, Mariana A. Reyes, Tony Kuo and Noel C. Barragan
Comorbidity of Type 2 Diabetes and Dementia among Hospitalized Patients in Los Angeles County: Hospitalization Outcomes and Costs, 2019–2021
Reprinted from: *Diabetology* 2023, 4, 52, doi:10.3390/diabetology4040052 62

Bismark Owusu-Afriyie, Theresa Gende, Martin Tapilas, Nicholas Zimbare and Jeffrey Kewande
Patients' Perspective on Barriers to Utilization of a Diabetic Retinopathy Screening Service
Reprinted from: *Diabetology* 2023, 4, 33, doi:10.3390/diabetology4030033 76

Marija Rogoznica, Dražen Perica, Barbara Borovac, Andrej Belančić and Martina Matovinović
Sexual Dysfunction in Female Patients with Type 2 Diabetes Mellitus—Sneak Peek on an Important Quality of Life Determinant
Reprinted from: *Diabetology* 2023, 4, 46, doi:10.3390/diabetology4040046 89

Jay H. Shubrook, Joshua J. Neumiller, Radica Z. Alicic, Tom Manley and Katherine R. Tuttle
Best Practices in the Use of Sodium–Glucose Cotransporter 2 Inhibitors in Diabetes and Chronic Kidney Disease for Primary Care
Reprinted from: *Diabetology* 2023, 4, 39, doi:10.3390/diabetology4040039 99

Marin Golčić and Andrej Belančić
Could Microbiome Be the Common Co-Denominator between Type 2 Diabetes and Pancreatic Cancer?
Reprinted from: *Diabetology* **2023**, *4*, 49, doi:10.3390/diabetology4040049 . . . . **111**

Andrej Belančić and Sanja Klobučar
Sodium-Glucose Co-Transporter 2 Inhibitors as a Powerful Cardioprotective and Renoprotective Tool: Overview of Clinical Trials and Mechanisms
Reprinted from: *Diabetology* **2023**, *4*, 22, doi:10.3390/diabetology4030022 . . . . **118**

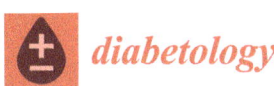

Article

Prevalence of Peripheral Arterial Disease and Principal Associated Risk Factors in Patients with Type 2 Diabetes Mellitus: The IDON-Peripheral Arterial Disease Study

Aliyanet Isamara Porcayo Ascencio *, Evangelina Morales Carmona, Jesús Morán Farías, Dulce Stephanie Guzmán Medina, Rebeca Galindo Salas and Leobardo Sauque Reyna

Instituto de Diabetes and Obesidad y Nutrición S.C., Cuernavaca 62250, Morelos, Mexico; evangelina.morales@insp.mx (E.M.C.); jchuymoran@gmail.com (J.M.F.); dradulcegm93@gmail.com (D.S.G.M.); rebecagalindo962@gmail.com (R.G.S.); leobardo.sauque@idonsc.com.mx (L.S.R.)
* Correspondence: personal.isamara.porcayo@gmail.com

Abstract: The principal purpose of this study is to determine the prevalence of peripheral arterial disease (PAD), as well as the principal associated risk factors, in patients registered in the IDON-PAD database. PAD is a condition characterized by the narrowing or blockage of arteries in the body's extremities due to plaque buildup, leading to reduced blood flow and tissue ischemia. While PAD primarily affects the lower extremities, it can lead to symptoms such as intermittent claudication and, in severe cases, ulcers and amputations. Risk factors for PAD are numerous and cumulative, including smoking, age over 50, type 2 diabetes mellitus, and hypertension. The prevalence of PAD increases with age, with rates ranging from 2.5% in those over 50 to 60% in those over 85, varying by ethnicity and study population. Diabetic patients face a higher risk of PAD-related complications and have lower success rates with revascularization procedures. The diagnosis of PAD traditionally relied on physical examination and symptoms, but the Ankle–Brachial Index is now a standard diagnostic tool due to its non-invasive nature and reliability. In Mexico, the prevalence of PAD is estimated at 10%, with significant risk factors being the duration of diabetes, hypertension, hypertriglyceridemia, and smoking. Notably, 70% of PAD cases are asymptomatic, emphasizing the importance of proactive screening. This study aimed to determine the prevalence of PAD and associated risk factors in diabetic patients aged 40 and above. The prevalence was found to be 11.2%, with high-risk waist circumference, elevated triglycerides, positive Edinburgh questionnaire, and weak pulses as significant predictors. The detection and management of PAD in diabetic patients require a comprehensive approach, including lifestyle modifications and regular screenings. Prevention strategies should focus on controlling risk factors, including obesity, hypertension, and dyslipidemia. In conclusion, PAD is a prevalent yet underdiagnosed condition in diabetic patients, necessitating proactive screening and comprehensive management to mitigate associated risks and improve patient outcomes. The principal limitation of this study is that, as it uses a cross-sectional methodology and is not an experimental study, although we can establish the prevalence of PAD as well as the associated risk factors, we cannot define causality or determine the hazard ratio for each of these factors. Special thanks to Dr. Leobardo Sauque Reyna and all participants for their contribution to this research.

Keywords: peripheral arterial disease (PAD); vascular non-traumatic amputation; type 2 diabetes mellitus; Ankle–Brachial Index (ABI); cross-sectional study; Morelos; México

1. Introduction

Peripheral arterial disease (PAD) is a syndrome characterized by a multifactorial etiology that manifests as stenosis or obstruction of the arterial lumen (excluding coronary and cerebral arteries) by an atheroma plaque that originates in the intima and proliferates within the lumen, causing hemodynamic changes in blood flow that diminish the perfusion pressure and generate local and distal tissue and organ ischemia.

In medical practice, the arterial obstruction of the lower extremities manifests as the presence of pain in the legs induced by walking—known as intermittent claudication—as well as paleness that, in critical stages, can cause ulcers and non-traumatic amputations that affect patients' quality of life [1,2].

The origin of the PAD is multifactorial, and its development includes multiple cardiovascular risk factors. The principal factors are cumulative, and when they coexist with factors, such as smoking, age of 50 years or older, type 2 diabetes mellitus T2DM, and hypertension, the severity of PAD increases [3].

The prevalence in patients over 50 years old is 2.5% and increases to 14.5% in patients over 70 years old. In the meta-analysis conducted by Vitalis A et al. [4] examining the prevalence of PAD across different ethnicities, a higher prevalence was found in African Americans and patients with type 2 diabetes mellitus (T2DM). In the latter group, the prevalence was up to four times higher compared to patients without diabetes. Similarly, in the study conducted by Cacoub P et al. in a French population at high risk (N = 5679), a 28% overall prevalence of PAD was observed. This contrasts with the 38% prevalence in the subgroup with the highest cardiovascular risk (subjects with a clinical history of atherothrombotic events) [5].

The prevalence of PAD in patients over 55 years old ranges from 3 to 29%, where the prevalence increases with age and is up to 60% in patients over 85 years old. The gap between these data is associated with ethnicity or race, the type of study population (higher or lower risk), and the methodology used to diagnose PAD [6].

The prognosis of PAD in patients with T2DM is less favorable than in patients without T2DM, as diabetic patients have a lower probability of success with revascularization and major cardiovascular morbimortality once PAD is present, as described in the article by Nativel M. et al. [7].

PAD can be diagnosed based on examination (skin color changes, cold extremities, and weak pulses) and symptoms (intermittent claudication and sensitivity alterations) [8], but the Ankle–Brachial Index (ABI) is now considered a standardized diagnostic method. It is a technique with the advantage of being non-invasive and painful, and it has acceptable precision, confidence, and reproducibility [9].

While information about PAD in the Latin American population is limited, we know that the prevalence of PAD in this group is around 12.5% [10].

In Mexico, the study performed by Buitrón-Granados L et al. [11]. followed a cross-sectional methodology and enrolled 400 patients who attended a first-level medical IMSS unit in Mexico City. They gathered information about previous medical history of T2DM, smoking, and hypertension, as well as laboratory variables and ABI index measurement (diagnostic cut point index of <0.9) with Doppler Ultrasound equipment (Doppler Versadopp@ 1000, Medzer Inc., Wilmington, DE, USA). At the end of the study, the global prevalence of PAD was 10% (14% in men and 8.4% in women). It stands out that the principal risk factors found were the duration of diabetes, the presence of hypertension, hypertriglyceridemia, and smoking. Just 30% of the patients with PAD had symptoms, while 70% were asymptomatic.

It is also known that both conditions (PAD and T2DM), alone and together, represent major public health issues and that both are considered cardiovascular risk factors. Many epidemiological studies have reported that patients with PAD have greater cardiovascular morbidity and mortality compared with patients without PAD [11,12]; on the other hand, it is well-known that patients with T2DM have a two-fold increase in cardiovascular risk for macrovascular events (myocardial infarction, stroke, and cardiovascular death) compared with the diabetic population [13,14].

PAD is considered an underdiagnosed condition due to a significant percentage of patients being asymptomatic. It is estimated that only 9% to 11% of patients report classic symptoms and, in a considerably high percentage of patients, the diagnosis is also delayed and is made when there is already severe tissue damage, ulcers, and/or amputation in the feet or pelvic limbs [15].

The poor detection of PAD, especially in asymptomatic populations, suggests that many patients will not receive appropriate treatment, particularly the management of peripheral arterial disease, as a cardiovascular risk factor, similar to the case for hypercholesterolemia and systemic arterial hypertension [16].

Regarding the incidence of PAD, a study by Hooi JD et al., which involved a 7.2-year follow up of a cohort of 2327 asymptomatic subjects in the Netherlands with the risk factors, revealed that the main factors increasing the risk of developing PAD are smoking, hypertension, and T2DM. This incidence study also emphasized the role of these factors in the cumulative risk [17].

A study by Rachael L. Morley et al. examined a population with a positive diagnosis of PAD, where 95% of patients had at least one of the risk factors, such as smoking and/or diabetes. Age was another significant risk factor, as in a population of 2174 patients studied, it was observed that the risk of developing PAD increased by 1% from 40 to 49 years old and by 15% in patients over 70 years old [18].

Patients with diabetes have up to 5.9 times greater risk of experiencing a cardiovascular event, as well as an added risk of developing PAD, which negatively impacts the functionality and quality of life of those who suffer from it. Patients with type 2 diabetes and PAD have a three to six times increased risk of experiencing a myocardial infarction [19].

Due to the high likelihood of developing PAD in patients with T2DM and the negative impact this has on their quality of life, the timely detection, treatment, and management of PAD as a cardiovascular risk factor are paramount for patients diagnosed with PAD. The ABI is the most widely used method for the diagnosis of PAD, as most patients may be asymptomatic [12].

Peripheral arterial disease in patients with diabetes is paramount in Mexico for several critical reasons. First, Mexico is experiencing a significant rise in the prevalence of diabetes, with estimates suggesting that nearly 13 million adults are affected by the disease [20]. Second, diabetes significantly increases the risk of developing PAD, with diabetic individuals being up to four times more likely to develop PAD compared to their non-diabetic counterparts [21]. Third, PAD in diabetic patients is associated with a higher risk of cardiovascular events, including myocardial infarction and stroke [15]. Due to the significance of PAD in the population with T2DM and the scarcity of data, the purpose of this study was to determine the prevalence of PAD, as well as the main associated risk factors, in patients with T2DM receiving care at the IDON, which is a population inherently at higher cardiovascular risk.

The primary objective of this study was to calculate the prevalence of PAD in patients registered in the IDON-PAD database by measuring their ABI using automated equipment from February 2020 to October 2021 and to identify the principal risk factors associated with design strategies of prevention, early treatment, and improved prognosis of patients with T2DM that attend the Instituto de Diabetes, Obesidad y Nutrición S.C. IDON in Cuernavaca, Morelos.

2. Material and Methods

This was a descriptive, comparative, and cross-sectional study.

The object of study was the IDON-PAD secondary database, which has a record of 734 patients with type 2 diabetes mellitus with at least 6 months of evolution who were treated at the IDON. The purpose of this project was to describe the prevalence of PAD in patients with type 2 diabetes registered in the IDON-PAD database who were treated at the IDON, as well as the association of PAD with the main variables of interest as risk factors.

As a first procedure, a deliberate search was conducted for patients at the Institute of Diabetes, Obesity, and Nutrition, located in Cuernavaca, Morelos, México, who had been diagnosed with at least 6 months of the evolution of type 2 diabetes mellitus and were aged at least 40 years. Once these patients were identified, they were invited to participate, following a thorough reading and signing of the informed consent (IC). The diagnosis of type 2 diabetes mellitus was considered when the following criterion was met: a diagnosis in the medical record in at least the last 6 months or receiving antidiabetic treatment in the last 6 months. The diagnostic criteria for T2DM were considered according to the criteria recommended by the American Diabetes Association 2019 ADA: glycated hemoglobin A1C > 6.5%, fasting plasma glucose > 126 mg/dL, and random glucose > 200 mg/dL. The measurement of glucose and hemoglobin was carried out after a minimum fast of 8 h, according to the photocolorimetry method for plasma glucose [22].

Including patients aged 40 and above in this study offers a broader perspective on peripheral arterial disease across various age groups. This approach enhances our understanding of how the disease progresses over time and its prevalence at different life stages. By avoiding age restrictions, a more comprehensive and accurate portrayal of the disease in the general population can be achieved. Despite its lower prevalence in younger individuals, evidence suggests that peripheral arterial disease can manifest in adults as young as 55, indicating that it is not exclusive to older age groups. Studies consistently show a notable increase in the prevalence of the disease with age. This inclusive approach allows for a more precise examination of this trend and insight into disease progression. Given its role as a significant risk factor for severe cardiovascular events, like heart attacks and strokes, grasping its prevalence across diverse age brackets is crucial for crafting effective public health policies. The inclusion of individuals aged 40 and above in this study furnishes valuable insights for identifying high-risk populations and implementing timely preventive measures.

Once informed consent was obtained, patients' medical records were reviewed, clinical and laboratory information was updated, and a log of clinical laboratory variables was completed. Subsequently, upon reviewing the log of variables and applying applicable inclusion and exclusion criteria, the ABI was measured using the automated vasera 2000 method.

2.1. Population

The population was older than 40 years old and had a diagnosis of at least 6 months of T2DM evolution. Their data were obtained from the IDON-PAD secondary database and the second-level clinic (Instituto de Diabetes, Obesidad y Nutrición S.C.) in Cuernavaca, Morelos, during the time period from February 2020 to October 2021 if they met the relevant criteria.

2.2. Inclusion Criteria

Patients older than 40 years old.
Diagnosis of T2DM of at least 6 months of evolution.
Patients living in the state of Morelos, México.

2.3. Exclusion Criteria

Patients with incomplete information in the database (absence of 1 or more of the clinical and laboratory variables of interest).

2.4. Population Sample

Non-probabilistic convenience sampling was performed by taking all the records available in the IDON-PAD database that were found to be complete (all independent variables complete), met the inclusion criteria, and did not meet any of the exclusion criteria.

2.5. Data Collections Methods

No additional information was collected from the patients; only the information available in the IDON-PAD secondary database was utilized. The IDON-PAD database was created for research purposes, and patient information was collected after informed consent was obtained, such that the patients authorized the use of their personal and laboratory data. All variables were gathered from the patients' medical records.

2.6. Ethical Considerations

Before the procedures and collection of data from the participating subjects, the procedures were fully explained, and the informed consent form version 1.0, approved by the research ethics committee on 26 March 2020 and the research committee on 26 March 2020, was read.

This protocol was conducted in accordance with the provisions of the Regulation of the General Heath Law on research, Ministry of Health (1984), specifically in the following sections: Articles 14, 15, 16, 17, 18, 19, 21, 22, and 29. Furthermore, both the informed consent form and the process of obtaining informed consent were carried out in accordance with the Nuremberg Code, the Belmont Report, and the Helsinki Declaration [23].

2.7. Analysis of the Information

Once the complete and correct information was available for the objectives of this study, the population of the database was characterized. The clinical and demographic characteristics were described using descriptive statistics. Continuous variables are expressed as means ± standard deviation using mode and median, and dichotomous variables are expressed as relative frequencies, which were estimated using binomial logistic regression analysis.

The prevalence of peripheral arterial disease detected by ABI measurement was obtained according to the proportion of patients with an ABI of 0.9 compared to patients with a normal ABI (>0.9). This was calculated with a confidence interval of 95%, and the respective prevalence by age and sex was also calculated.

To compare the qualitative variables between the patients with positive peripheral arterial disease vs. the patients with negative peripheral arterial disease, the chi-square test was first used and, for the variables with low frequency, Fisher's test was used to compare the means and obtain the p-value.

To identify the risk factors associated with PAD in the study population, a multiple logistic regression model was performed. Before the multiple logistic regression was performed, the relationship between the dependent variable and the independent variables was explored through simple logistic regressions. In addition, the correlations between the qualitative and quantitative independent variables were analyzed. For quantitative variables that met the Kolmogorov–Smirnov hypothesis test of a non-normal parametric distribution of the data, Spearman's coefficient was used, and for normally distributed variables, Pearson's coefficient was used.

In the single and multiple regressions, the quantitative variables were analyzed as categorical variables, with categories constructed according to their clinical relevance, as shown in the next table. The age variable was classified by decades, and the high variable was in increments of 20. For the somatometry variables—body mass index kg/m^2 (BMI), waist circumference, waist–hip ratio, and fat percentage—the WHO classification of risk was used [20]. We decided to add the waist–hip ratio as a variable instead of hip circumference for classification by sex [20], according to the WHO. The percentage of fat was also classified according to sex, including sub-optimal weight, slightly overweight, overweight, and obese. For the blood pressure variables (systolic and diastolic), the AHA [24] classification was used. Laboratory variables, such as HDL cholesterol and triglycerides, were classified according to AHA recommendations [24]. The glycosylated hemoglobin variable was classified according to the recommendations of the ADA [25]. Basal fasting glucose was classified as control, normal–high, slightly high, or very high. The estimated glomerular filtration rate variable, calculated using mdrd, was categorized according to the Chronic Kidney Disease Foundation's classification [26]. The variables of weight, heart rate, creatinine, total cholesterol, and LDL cholesterol were classified by quartiles as, based on the frequencies, if they were classified by statistical relevance, there would be groups with very low frequencies, which would weaken the statistical analysis.

In the Table 1 below, the way in which quantitative variables were categorized for analysis is shown.

Table 1. Categorization of quantitative variables.

Variable	Categories
Years (y)	• 40–49 years old • 50–59 years old • 60–69 years old • >70 years old
Height (cm)	• 1.30–1.49 cm • 1.50–1.59 cm • 1.60–1.69 cm • 1.70–1.79 cm
Weight (kg)	• Q1 60.9 kg • Q2 70.75 kg • Q3 80.82 kg • Q4 167.1 kg
IMC (kg/m^2)	• Low and normal weight (<24.9) • Overweight (25.0–29.9) • Obesity (>30.0)
Waist circumference (cm)	• Low risk (F: <80 cm, M: <95cm) • High risk (F: 80–88 cm, M: 95–101 cm) • Very high risk (F: >88 cm, M: >101 cm)
Waist–hip index	• Low–normal (F: <0.84, M: <0.94) • High (F: >0.84, M: >0.94)
Body fat (%)	• Sub-optimal (F: 20.9, M: >15.9) • Slightly overweight (F: 21–25.9, M: 16–20.9) • Overweight (F: 26–31.9, M: 21–24.9) • Obesity (F: >32, M: >25)
Systolic blood pressure (mm/hg)	• Normal (<120 mm/hg) • High (120–129 mm/hg) • Arterial hypertension 1 (130–139 mm/hg) • Arterial hypertension 2 (>140 mm/hg)
Diastolic blood pressure (mm/hg)	• Hypotension (<80 mm/hg) • Normotension (80–89 mm/hg) • Hypertension (>90 mm/hg)
Heart rate (bpm)	• Q1: 69 l pm • Q2: 75 l pm • Q3: 82 l pm • Q4: 151 l pm
Serum creatinine (mg/dL)	• Q1: 0.68 mg/dL • Q2: 0.8 mg/dL • Q3: 1.0 mg/dL • Q4: 11.24 mg/dL
Total cholesterol (mg/dL)	• Q1: 146 mg/dL • Q2: 179 mg/dL • Q3: 208 mg/dL • Q4: 386 mg/dL

Table 1. *Cont.*

Variable	Categories
High-density cholesterol (mg/dL)	• Low (<40 mg/dL) • Normal (40–60 mg/dL) • High (>60 mg/dL)
Low-density cholesterol (mg/dL)	• Q1: 36.4 mg/dL • Q2: 44 mg/dL • Q3: 52.4 mg/dL • Q4: 182 mg/dL
Serum triglycerides (mg/dL)	• 0–99 mg/dL • 100–149 mg/dL • 150–199 mg/dL • 200–299 mg/dL • >300 mg/dL
Glycated hemoglobin (%)	• 5–6.9% • 7–7.9% • 8–8.9% • 9–9.9% • >10%
Fasting basal glucose (mg/dL)	• 0–99 mg/dL • 100–149 mg/dL • 150–199 mg/dL • >200 mg/dL
Estimated glomerular filtration rate (mL/min/1.73 m^2)	• Normal (>90 mL/min/1.73 m^2) • Low decrease (60–89 mL/min/1.73 m^2) • Moderate decrease (30–59 mL/min/1.73 m^2) • Severe decrease (<30 mL/min/1.73 m^2)

F: feminine sex. M: masculine sex. BMI: body mass index.

Finally, the crude contribution of the independent variables as predictor variables was evaluated, all the analyzable variables were analyzed using a multiple logistic regression model with PAD as the dependent variable, and a multiple logistic regression was subsequently performed that was adjusted for the variables with the highest statistically significant correlation coefficients, according to the correlation analysis carried out between the independent variables and the dependent variable.

All *p*-values were calculated with two tails and were considered significant if they were less than 0.05. To find out the strength and direction of the association between the independent variables and the PAD, the odds ratios and their 95% confidence intervals were calculated using the Stata 16 program.

To guarantee that the research protocol and the techniques used to keep patient data confidential were certified, the protocol was sent to the Research Ethics Committee of the National Institute of Public Health for review and approval.

3. Results

In Table 2, we can observe the baseline characteristics of the qualitative variables of the patients. In Table 3, we have the baseline characteristics of the quantitative variables of the patients, where we observe that the mean of characteristics is an age og 61 years, with a BMI of 28.

Table 2. Description of the qualitative variables.

Qualitative Variable	Frequency (N = 632)	Percentage (%)
Positive PAD	71	11
Feminine sex	373	59
Masculine sex	259	41
Smoking	150	24
Systemic arterial hypertension	337	53
Dyslipidemia	308	49
Cardiovascular event	59	9
Acute myocardial infarction	29	5
Non-traumatic vascular amputation	13	2
Cerebral vascular disease	16	3
Positive diabetic retinopathy	75	12
Positive eye surgery	92	15
Laser treatment treatment	75	12
Antihypertensive treatment	321	51
Lipid-lowering treatment	270	43
Basal insulin treatment	147	23
Intermediate insulin treatment	72	11
Fast insulin treatment	16	3
Premixed insulin treatment	24	4
Oral hypoglycemic agent treatment	562	89
Injectable hypoglycemic agents	5	1
Premixed insulin + glp1 treatment	19	3
Antiplatelet agent treatment	58	9
Anticoagulant treatment	2	1
Proteinuria	94	15
Neuropathic pain	41	7
Alteration of sensitivity in pelvic limbs	151	24
Positive Edinburgh questionnaire	71	11
Signs or symptoms of positive PAD	51	8
Changes in color in pelvic extremities	23	4
Claudication	13	2
Weak pulses in pelvic extremities	4	1
Dryness in pelvic extremities	4	1
Presence of ulcers in pelvic extremities	7	1

PAD: peripheral arterial disease.

Table 3. Description of the quantitative variables.

Quantitative Variable	Mean	Minimum	Maximum
Years	61 ± 10	40	90
Height (cm)	159 ± 6	136	185
Weight (kg)	72 ± 16	41.4	167.1
BMI (kg/m^2)	28 ± 5	17.5	55.2
Waist circumference (cm)	96 ± 12	47	154
Hip circumference (cm)	101 ± 12	42	145
Body fat (%)	33 ± 10	9.1	59
Diastolic blood pressure (mm/hg)	75 ± 13	43	178
Systolic blood pressure (mm/hg)	127 ± 21	79	218
Heart rate (bpm)	76 ± 12	47	151
Serum creatinine (mg/dL)	0.96 ± 0.75	0.29	11.24
Total cholesterol (mg/dL)	177 ± 50	69	386
High-density cholesterol (mg/dL)	46 ± 15	19.3	182
Low-density cholesterol (mg/dL)	111 ± 42	24.6	242.9
Serum triglycerides (mg/dL)	180 ± 119	33.6	979
Glycated hemoglobin (%)	8.6 ± 3	5	17.8
Fasting basal glucose (mg/dL)	158 ± 72	63.3	570
Estimated glomerular filtration rate (mL/min/1.73 m^2)	82.3 ± 27	4.3	158.8

BMI: body mass index.

In Table 4, we can observe the proportion of patients according to glycated hemoglobin levels, finding the population to be polarized, with the highest proportion of patients in the range of 5–6.9%, followed by a glycated hemoglobin > 10%.

Table 4. Frequency of patients according to glycated hemoglobin results.

Glycosylated Hemoglobin Group	Frequency (N = 632)	Percentage (%)
5–6.9%	178	28.2
7–7.9%	139	22.0
8–9.9%	83	13.1
9–9.9%	72	11.4
>10%	160	25.3

3.1. PAD Prevalence

The prevalence of PAD was 11.2%, with a total of 71 patients, of whom 40 (56.3%) were female and 31 (43.7%) were male.

3.2. Comparative Groups of Qualitative Variables

The variables that had a statistically significant difference between both groups were the presence of systemic arterial hypertension and the presence of a previous vascular event or atherosclerotic cardiovascular disease (specifically, non-traumatic vascular amputation), history of eye surgery, antihypertensive treatment, treatment with insulin, the presence of proteinuria, positive sensitivity alteration, positive Edinburgh questionnaire, the presence of signs or symptoms of peripheral arterial disease, color changes, limp gait, weak pulses, dryness, and the presence of ulcers (see Table 5). The difference in proportions of the statistically significant qualitative variables between the positive PAD and the negative PAD groups was then observed.

Table 5. Comparison of the qualitative variables with negative PAD vs. positive PAD.

Variables	Positive PAD Ratio (T = 71)	Negative PAD Ratio (T = 561)	Chi-Square	Fisher's Exact Test
Female sex	0.56	0.59	0.626	
Smoking	0.28	0.23	0.351	
Systemic arterial hypertension	0.65	0.52	0.040 *	
Dyslipidemia	0.41	0.50	0.158	
Previous vascular event or atherosclerotic vascular disease	0.18	0.08	0.006 *	
Acute myocardial infarction	0.07	0.04		0.359
Non-traumatic vascular amputation	0.06	0.02		0.048 *
Cerebrovascular ischemic event	0.06	0.02		0.094
Diabetic retinopathy	0.18	0.11	0.075	
History of eye surgery	0.28	0.13	0.001 *	
Eye laser treatment	0.20	0.11	0.471	
Antihypertensive treatment	0.66	0.49	0.006 *	
Lipid-lowering treatment	0.46	0.42	0.497	
Oral hypoglycemic treatment	0.86	0.89	0.391	
Insulin treatment	0.57	0.39	0.003 *	
Injectable hypoglycemic treatment	0.00	0.01		1.000
Antiplatelet agent treatment	0.17	0.08	0.017	
Anticoagulant treatment	0.00	0.00		1.000
Proteinuria	0.27	0.13	0.003 *	
Neuropathic pain	0.10	0.06		0.206
Possible neuropathic pain	0.13	0.07	0.063	
Sensitivity altered in pelvic members	0.44	0.21	0.000 *	
Positive Edinburgh questionnaire	0.28	0.09	0.000 *	
Signs and symptoms of positive PAD	0.18	0.07	0.001 *	
Color changes	0.10	0.03		0.009 *
Faltering gate	0.03	0.02		0.648
Weak pulses	0.04	0.00		0.005 *
Dry skin	0.00	0.01		1.000
Ulcers	0.01	0.01		0.568

PAD: peripheral arterial disease.

3.3. Comparative Groups of Quantitative Variables

The variables that had a statistically significant difference between the means are shown in Table 6. We can see that patients with positive PAD had a higher mean age, serum creatinine, waist circumference, hip circumference, and systolic blood pressure than patients with negative PAD, while PAD-positive patients had a lower glomerular filtration rate than patients with negative PAD.

Table 6. Comparison of the quantitative variables with negative PAD vs. positive PAD.

Variables	Mean PAD Positive	Mean PAD Negative	Kolmogorov–Smirnov Test	Student's t-Test	Mann–Whitney U Test
Height (cm)	159.9	159.7	0.001	0.8755	
Age (years)	65.4	60.7	0.143		0.003 *
Weight (kg)	74.4	72.3	0.026	0.6370	
Body mass index	28.8	28.3	0.000	0.8590	
Waist circumference (cm)	99.3	95.6	0.062		0.0138 *
Hip circumference (cm)	103.8	100.7	0.014	0.0415 *	
Average of fat (%)	32.6	32.4	0.346		0.848
Systolic blood pressure (mm/Hg)	135.5	125.9	0.000	0.0038 *	
Diastolic blood pressure (mm/Hg)	73.9	74.6	0.004	0.9069	
Heart rate (bpm)	77.6	75.9	0.001	0.6020	
Serum creatinine (mg/dL)	1.20	0.93	0.000	0.0006 *	
Total cholesterol (mg/dL)	186.6	176.6	0.178		0.1212
High-density cholesterol (mg/dL)	48.7	46.1	0.000	0.8009	
Low-density cholesterol (mg/dL)	114.1	110.5	0.322		0.5620
Triglycerides (mg/dL)	180.6	180.1	0.000	0.3610	
Glycosylated hemoglobin (%)	8.6	8.6	0.000	0.5921	
Basal glucose (mg/dL)	165.1	157.5	0.000	0.4457	
Glomerular filtration rate (mL/min/1.73 m^2)	69.2	84.0	0.009	0.0000 *	

PAD: peripheral arterial disease.

The correlations between the dependent variable PAD and the qualitative independent variables as shown in Table 7 were evaluated, with statistically significant correlations found in the following variables: the presence of systemic arterial hypertension, history of laser treatment, history of eye surgery, treatment with antihypertensive drugs, intermediate insulin treatment, treatment with antiplatelet agents, alteration of sensitivity, Edinburgh questionnaire, signs or symptoms suggestive of PAD, changes in limb coloration, and weak pulses in pelvic extremities.

Table 7. Correlation between the dependent variable PAD and the qualitative independent variables.

Variable	Frequency	Correlation	Confidence Interval	p
Systemic arterial hypertension	337	1.70	1.02–2.85	0.042
Cardiovascular event	59	2.50	1.28–4.91	0.007
Non-traumatic vascular amputation	13	3.66	1.09–12.21	0.035
Laser eye treatment	75	2.01	1.05–3.82	0.033
Eye surgery	92	2.66	1.50–4.72	0.001
Antihypertensive treatment	321	2.05	1.22–3.44	0.007
Intermediate insulin treatment	72	2.62	1.40–4.88	0.002
Antiplatelet agent treatment	58	2.27	1.14–4.54	0.019
Alteration of sensitivity in pelvic limbs	151	2.84	1.70–4.74	0.000
Positive Edinburgh questionnaire	71	3.92	2.16–7.08	0.000
Signs and symptoms of PAD	51	3.08	1.55–6.12	0.001
Changes in the color of the pelvic limbs	23	3.72	1.47–9.39	0.005
Weak pulses in pelvic limbs	4	24.70	2.53–240.84	0.006

PAD: peripheral arterial disease.

3.4. Positive Cases by Age

Among our population, 65.1% (411) were between 55 and 70 years old, 14.4% (91) were over 70 years old, and 20.5% (130) were less than 55 years old.

In Figure 1, we can see that the largest volume of positive cases for PAD was found in the 60- to 69-year-old group, with 39.4% (28), followed by 28.1% (20) for the 70- to 79-year-old group, 17% (12) for the group from 50 to 59 years, 8.5% (6) for the group from 80 to 90 years, and, finally, 7% (5) for the group from 40 to 49 years. The highest proportion of positive cases of PAD was found in the group of 80 to 90 years at a proportion of 0.28.

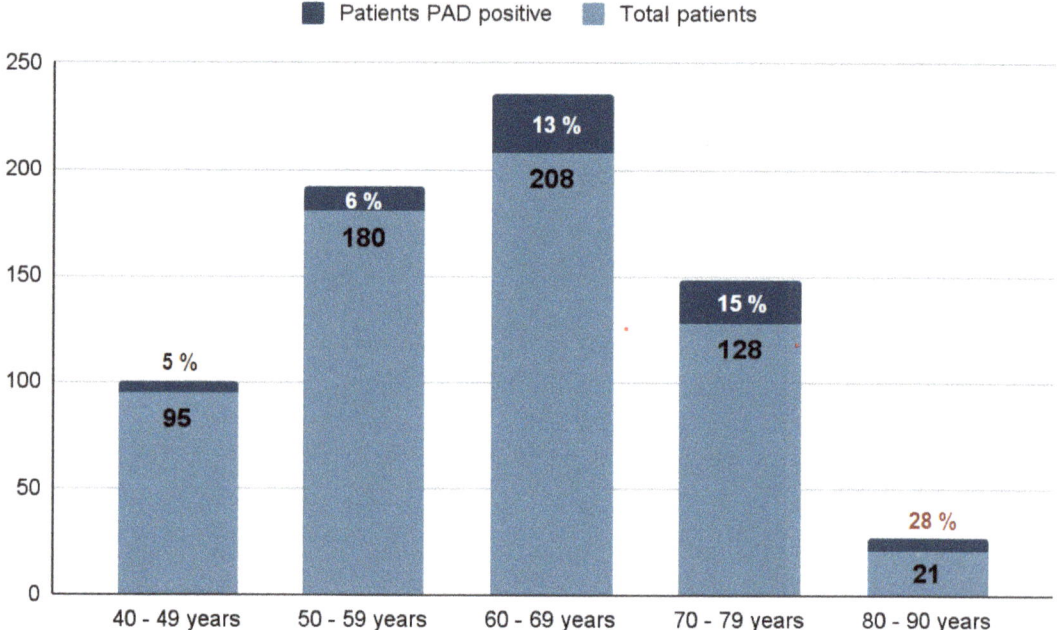

Figure 1. Frequency and rate of PAD (+) by age group.

3.5. Multiple Logistic Regression

Initially, a crude multivariate logistic regression was run using all the independent variables with the dependent variable; however, as it is a crude multiple logistic regression, multicollinearity between the independent variables was present, which reduced its predictive capacity. Therefore, a multivariate logistic regression was subsequently run that did not analyze the strongly correlated variables (see Table 8), and it was adjusted according to the correlations between the independent variables that, in the simple regression, showed a statistically significant correlation with the dependent variable. We can observe that the variables with statistical relevance were high waist circumference, very high waist circumference, triglycerides between 150 and 199 mg/dL, positive Edinburgh questionnaire, and weak pulses in the lower extremities during the examination.

With the other variables held constant, subjects with a waist circumference classified as high risk (F: 80–88 cm, M: 95–101 cm) were 4.58 times more likely to present PAD, and subjects with a waist circumference classified as very high risk (F: >88 cm, M: >102 cm) were up to 3.39 times more likely to have PAD than patients with a low-risk waist circumference. Patients with serum triglycerides between 150 and 199 mg/dL were 3.14 times more likely to present PAD than those patients with serum triglycerides < 100 mg/dL. Patients who presented a positive Edinburgh questionnaire were 3.35 times more likely to present PAD than patients who reported a negative Edinburgh questionnaire. Patients who presented weak pulses in the lower extremities during the physical examination were 25.49 times more likely to present PAD than those who presented pulses of adequate intensity during the physical examination.

Table 8. Multiple logistic regression model adjusted for the correlation of independent variables strongly associated with the dependent variable.

PAD Positive	Odds Ratio	Std. Err.	p	Confidence Interval
Male sex	0.78	0.26	0.443	0.41–1.48
50–59 years	0.88	0.52	0.823	0.27–2.80
60–69 years	1.56	0.88	0.430	0.52–4.70
>70 years	1.83	1.10	0.315	0.56–5.94
High-risk waist circumference	4.58	2.41	1.004	1.63–12.85
Very-high-risk waist circumference	3.39	1.90	0.029	1.13–10.18
Fat percentage in slightly overweight	2.00	1.66	0.404	0.39–10.14
Fat percentage in overweight	1.29	1.00	0.738	0.29–5.86
Fat percentage in obesity	1.03	0.78	0.964	0.24–4.50
Quartile 2 heart rate	0.89	0.36	1.767	0.40–1.96
Quartile 3 heart rate	0.88	0.38	0.768	0.38–2.06
Quartile 4 heart rate	1.56	0.61	0.257	0.72–3.36
Systemic hypertension arterial	1.00	0.58	1.000	0.32–3.11
Cardiovascular event	1.17	0.56	0.745	0.46–2.99
Mon-traumatic vascular amputation	1.97	1.68	0.425	0.37–10.43
Eye laser treatment	1.20	0.52	0.667	0.52–2.81
Eye surgery treatment	1.93	0.78	0.104	0.87–4.24
Antihypertensive treatment	1.22	0.71	0.727	0.40–3.79
Intermediate insulin treatment	1.74	0.68	0.159	0.81–3.75
Antiplatelet treatment	1.99	0.85	0.106	0.86–4.60
Triglycerides 100–149 mg/dL	1.27	0.66	0.637	0.46–3.50
Triglycerides 150–199 mg/dL	3.15	1.59	0.023	1.17–8.48
Triglycerides 200–299 mg/dL	2.06	1.13	0.185	0.71–6.02
Triglycerides > 300 mg/dL	1.61	1.06	0.467	0.45–5.82
Mild chronic kidney disease	1.35	0.50	0.412	0.66–2.79
Moderate chronic kidney disease	1.61	0.73	0.290	0.66–3.92
Severe chronic kidney disease	1.61	0.97	0.428	0.50–5.24
Sensitivity altered	1.52	0.50	0.202	0.80–2.91
Positive Edinburgh questionnaire	3.36	1.18	0.001	1.69–6.69
Signs and symptoms of PAD	0.66	0.47	0.560	0.17–2.63
Symptom color change	3.78	3.25	0.122	0.70–20.35
Symptoms of weak pulses	25.49	39.56	0.037	1.22–533.82

PAD: peripheral arterial disease, Std. Err: standard error.

4. Discussion

This study revealed the prevalence of PAD among diabetic patients to be 11.2%, which is consistent with previous findings in the Mexican population [27]. This underscores the significant comorbidities among these patients, with systemic arterial hypertension, dyslipidemia, and smoking being prevalent risk factors [28], as well as highlights the complex interplay between diabetes and other cardiovascular risk factors, emphasizing the need for comprehensive management strategies [28].

The people in this study varied, with some being larger but having their blood pressure and LDL cholesterol relatively under control. However, many struggled with blood sugar control. This tells us that we cannot just focus on heart issues when treating diabetes; we need a more comprehensive approach to achieve better outcomes for everyone.

It is surprising that only 8% of patients showed signs of having PAD, meaning that many cases could go unnoticed [27]. This reminds us of the importance of having a suspicious mindset in medical consultations and conducting thorough physical examinations, especially given that many PAD patients do not show obvious symptoms. Therefore, we need to make more efforts to detect PAD early and prevent future complications.

People with PAD are at higher risk of serious problems, such as heart attacks or amputations, as well as eye problems [7]. This indicates that diabetes-related vascular issues affect not just the heart but the whole body, highlighting the importance of detecting these problems early and treating them properly. It is vital to focus on maintaining a healthy weight, controlling triglyceride levels, and conducting comprehensive physical examinations in people with diabetes to detect PAD as early as possible and improve daily life and also reduce the risk of serious complications, like foot ulcers or amputations.

Prevention strategies will have to be designed to ensure that patients have the least associated comorbidities, controlling weight, waist circumference, blood pressure levels, and laboratory tests, such as cholesterol (total, HDL, LDL), triglycerides, and serum creatinine.

With the results of this study, it is not possible to accept the hypothesis that the main risk factors associated with PAD are positive smoking and advanced age. When constructing the correlation matrix, we noticed that the sample is probably insufficient for a model with so many variables, such as those included in the database, in addition to the fact that, when trying to classify them, there were categories with very low frequencies, which forced us to classify them by quartiles and not clinical relevance.

5. Conclusions

Peripheral arterial disease is a prevalent and underdiagnosed disease in first- and second-level care. It was found to have a prevalence of 11.2% in patients with type 2 diabetes mellitus who were seen in a second-level care clinic.

The main associated risk factors were waist circumference with high risk (4.5 more times); waist circumference with very high risk (3.3 more times); serum triglycerides greater than 150 mg/dL and less than 199 mg/dL (3.1 more times); and positive Edinburgh questionnaire (3.3 more times).

The main sign that we can observe in patients with positive PAD is the positive Edinburgh questionnaire, as this procedure should be carried out in all visits of patients with type 2 diabetes mellitus.

It is essential to actively search for signs or symptoms indicative of peripheral arterial disease in all patients with type 2 diabetes mellitus during regular medical consultations, as well as to incorporate the Edinburgh questionnaire into each visit. Additionally, regular measurement of the ABI should be encouraged for the early detection of PAD.

Encouraging healthy lifestyle habits among patients with T2DM is crucial to prevent and control the associated comorbidities. Keeping these conditions within control targets can significantly reduce the risk of both macrovascular and microvascular complications.

Author Contributions: Conceptualization; A.I.P.A., E.M.C. and L.S.R., methodology; A.I.P.A., E.M.C. and L.S.R., software; A.I.P.A. and E.M.C., validation; L.S.R. and E.M.C., formal analysis: A.I.P.A., E.M.C. and L.S.R., investigation; A.I.P.A., J.M.F., D.S.G.M., R.G.S., resources; L.S.R., data curation; A.I.P.A., E.M.C. and L.S.R., writing—original draft preparation; A.I.P.A., E.M.C. and L.S.R., writing—review and editing; A.I.P.A. and L.S.R., visualization, A.I.P.A., supervision, E.M.C. and L.S.R., project administration; A.I.P.A. and L.S.R., funding acquisition; L.S.R. All authors have read and agreed to the published version of the manuscript.

Funding: This research was funded by the Instituto de Diabetes, Obesidad and Nutrición S.C, in Cuernavaca Morelos.

Institutional Review Board Statement: The study was conducted in accordance with the Declaration of Helsinki, and approved by Ethics Committee of RIO MAYO MEDICA, local version No. 1.0 8MX and date of approval 14 feb for studies involving humans.

Informed Consent Statement: Informed consent was obtained from all subjects involved in the study.

Data Availability Statement: The available informationfrom the complete database used in this study is on Zenodo, with the DOI: 10.5281/zenodo.11176030.

Acknowledgments: Thanks to Leobardo Sauque Reyna, director of the Institute of Diabetes, Obesity, and Nutrition, for giving us all the support and tools to make this research possible. Thank you to all the participants and subjects of the sample who gladly contributed to the research. Thanks to the entire multidisciplinary team that contributed in very specific and varied ways to generate this scientific research.

Conflicts of Interest: The authors declare no conflict of interest.

References

1. Regensteiner, J.G.; Hiatt, W.R.; Coll, J.R.; Criqui, M.H.; Treat-Jacobson, D.; McDermott, M.M.; Hirsch, A.T. The impact of peripheral arterial disease on health-related quality of life in the Peripheral Arterial Disease Awareness, Risk, and Treatment: New Resources for Survival (PARTNERS) Program. *Vasc. Med. Lond. Engl.* **2008**, *13*, 15–24. [CrossRef]
2. Ouriel, K. Peripheral arterial disease. *Lancet* **2001**, *13*, 57–64. [CrossRef]
3. Norgren, L.; Hiatt, W.; Dormandy, J.; Nehler, M.; Harris, K.; Fowkes, F.; TASC II Working Group. Inter-Society Consensus for the Management of Peripheral Arterial Disease (TASC II). *J. Vasc. Surg.* **2007**, *45*, 5–67. [CrossRef]
4. Antonios, V.; Gregory, Y.H.L.; Mark, K.; Rajiv, K.V.; Alena, S. Ethnic differences in the prevalence of peripheral arterial disease: A systematic review and meta-analysis. *Expert Rev. Cardiovasc. Ther.* **2017**, *15*, 328–338. [CrossRef]
5. Cacoub, P.; Cambou, J.-P.; Kownator, S.; Belliard, J.-P.; Beregi, J.-P.; Branchereau, A.; Carpentier, P.; Léger, P.; Luizy, F.; Maïza, D.; et al. Prevalence of peripheral arterial disease inhigh-risk patients using ankle-brachial index in general practice: Across-sectional study. *Int. J. Clin. Pract.* **2009**, *63*, 63–70. [CrossRef]
6. Darling, J.; Bodewes, T.; Deery, S.; Guzman, R.; Wyers, M.; Hamdan, A.; Verhagen, H.J.; Schermerhorn, M.L. Outcomes after frst-time lower extremity revascularization for chronic limb-threatening ischemia between patients with and without diabetes. *Vasc. Surg.* **2018**, *67*, 59–69. [CrossRef]
7. Nativel, M.; Potier, L.; Alexandre, L.; Baillet-Blanco, L.; Ducasse, E.; Velho, G.; Marre, M.; Roussel, R.; Rigalleau, V.; Mohammedi, K. Lower extremity arterial disease in patients with diabetes: A contemporary narrative review. *Cardiovasc. Diabetol.* **2018**, *23*, 17–138. [CrossRef]
8. Burk, H. *Das Hunderttage-Stadion Entstehungsgeschichte des Bad Nauheimer Kunsteisstadions unter Colonel Paul R. Knight*; Stadt Bad Nauheim: Bad Nauheim, Germany, 1999.
9. Ko, S.; Bandyk, D. Interpretation and significance of ankle-brachial systolic pressure index. *Semin. Vasc. Surg.* **2013**, *26*, 86–94. [CrossRef] [PubMed]
10. Rosero, E.; Kane, K.; Clagett, G.; Timaran, C.H. A systematic review of the limitations and approaches to improve detection and management of peripheral arterial disease in Hispanics. *Vasc. Surg.* **2010**, *51*, 27–35. [CrossRef] [PubMed]
11. Buitrón-Granados, L.; Martínez-López, C.; Escobedo-de la Peña, J. Prevalence of peripheral arterial disease and related risk factors in an urban Mexican population. *Angiology* **2004**, *55*, 43–51. [CrossRef] [PubMed]
12. Newman, A.; Shemanski, L.; Manolio, T.; Cushman, M.; Mittelmark, M.; Polak, J.; Powe, N.R.; Siscovick, D. Ankle-arm index as a predictor of cardiovascular disease and mortality in the Cardiovascular Health Study. The Cardiovascular Health Study Group. *Arter. Vasc. Biol.* **1999**, *19*, 38–45.
13. Emerging Risk Factors Collaboration; Sarwar, N.; Gao, P.; Seshasai, S.R.; Gobin, R.; Kaptoge, S.; Di Angelantonio, E.; Ingelsson, E.; Lawlor, D.A.; Selvin, E.; et al. Diabetes mellitus, fasting blood glucose concentration, and risk of vascular disease: A collaborative meta-analysis of 102 prospective studies. *Lancet* **2010**, *375*, 15–22.
14. Resnick, H.; Lindsay, R.; McDermott, M.; Devereux, R.; Jones, K.; Fabsitz, R.; Howard, B.V. Relationship of high and low ankle brachial index to all-cause and cardiovascular disease mortality: The Strong Heart Study. *Circulation* **2004**, *17*, 109–733.
15. Hirsch, A.; Criqui, M.; Treat-Jacobson DRegensteiner, J.; Creager, M.; Olin, J.; Krook, S.; Krook, S.H.; Hunninghake, D.B.; Comerota, A.J.; Walsh, M.E.; et al. Peripheral arterial disease detection, awareness, and treatment in primary care. *JAMA* **2001**, *19*, 17–24. [CrossRef] [PubMed]
16. Rada, C.; Oummou, S.; Merzouk, F.; Amarir, B.; Boussabnia, G.; Bougrini, H.; Benzaroual, D.; Elkarimi, S.; Elhattaoui, M. Ankle-brachial index screening for peripheral artery disease in high cardiovascular risk patients. Prospective observational study of 370 asymptomatic patients at high cardiovascular risk. *J. Mal. Vasc.* **2016**, *41*, 353–357. [CrossRef]
17. Hooi, J.D.; Kester, A.D.; Stoffers, H.E.; Overdijk, M.M.; van Ree, J.W.; Knottnerus, J.A. Incidence of and risk factors for asymptomatic peripheral arterial occlusive disease: A longitudinal study. *Am. J. Epidemiol.* **2001**, *153*, 66–72. [CrossRef] [PubMed]
18. Morley, R.L.; Sharma, A.; Horsch, A.D.; Hinchliffe, R.J. Peripheral artery disease. *BMJ* **2018**, *360*, j5842. [CrossRef] [PubMed]
19. Zhang, X.; Ran, X.; Xu, Z.; Cheng, Z.; Shen, F.; Yu, Y.; Gao, L.; Chai, S.; Wang, C.; Liu, J.; et al. Epidemiological characteristics of lower extremity arterial disease in Chinese diabetes patients at high risk: A prospective, multicenter, cross-sectional study. *J. Diabetes Its Complicat.* **2018**, *32*, 150–156. [CrossRef] [PubMed]
20. American Diabetes Association. Standards of Medical Care in Diabetes. *Diabetes Care* **2019**, *42*, S13–S28.
21. Asociación Médica Mundial. Declaración de Helsinki de la AMM—Principios Éticos Para las Investigaciones Médicas en Seres Humanos. 2013. Available online: https://www.wma.net/es/policies-post/declaracion-de-la-amm-principios-eticos-para-las-investigaciones-medicas-en-seres-humanos/ (accessed on 13 April 2024).

22. WHO. The Use and Interpretation of Anthropometry. In *Physical Status: The Use of and Interpretation of Anthropometry*; Report of a WHO Expert Committee; WHO: Geneva, Switzerland, 1995.
23. Grundy, S.M.; Stone, N.J.; Bailey, A.L.; Beam, C.; Birtcher, K.K.; Blumenthal, R.S.; Braun, L.T.; de Ferranti, S.; Faiella-Tommasino, J.; Forman, D.E.; et al. AHA/ACC/AACVPR/AAPA/ABC/ACPM/ADA/AGS/APhA/ASPC/NLA/PCNA guideline on the management of blood cholesterol. *Am. Coll. Cardiol.* **2019**, *73*, 3168–3209. [CrossRef]
24. National Kidney Foundation. *Clinical Practice Guideline for the Evaluation and Management of Chronic Kidney Disease*; National Kidney Foundation, Inc.: New York, NY, USA, 2013; pp. 1–150.
25. Smith, A.B.; Maltais, S.; Kisilevsky, M.; Gagne, E. Peripheral Artery Disease: Epidemiology, Pathophysiology, and Clinical Presentation. *Curr. Cardiol. Rep.* **2022**, *24*, 1–12.
26. Fowkes, F.G.; Rudan, D.; Rudan, I.; Aboyans, V.; Denenberg, J.O.; McDermott, M.M.; Norman, P.E.; Sampson, U.K.; Williams, L.J.; Mensah, G.A.; et al. Comparison of global estimates of prevalence and risk factors for peripheral artery disease in 2000 and 2010: A systematic review and analysis. *Lancet* **2013**, *382*, 1329–1340. [CrossRef] [PubMed]
27. Selvin, E.; Erlinger, T.P. Prevalence of and risk factors for peripheral arterial disease in the United States: Results from the National Health and Nutrition Examination Survey, 1999–2000. *Circulation* **2004**, *110*, 738–743. [CrossRef] [PubMed]
28. Criqui, M.H.; Langer, R.D.; Fronek, A.; Feigelson, H.S.; Klauber, M.R.; McCann, T.J.; Browner, D. Mortality over a period of 10 years in patients with peripheral arterial disease. *N. Engl. J. Med.* **1992**, *326*, 381–386. [CrossRef] [PubMed]

Disclaimer/Publisher's Note: The statements, opinions and data contained in all publications are solely those of the individual author(s) and contributor(s) and not of MDPI and/or the editor(s). MDPI and/or the editor(s) disclaim responsibility for any injury to people or property resulting from any ideas, methods, instructions or products referred to in the content.

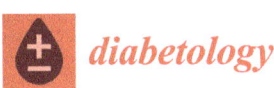

Article

Burden of Infected Diabetic Foot Ulcers on Hospital Admissions and Costs in a Third-Level Center

Roberto Da Ros [1,*], Roberta Assaloni [1], Andrea Michelli [1], Barbara Brunato [1], Enrica Barro [1], Marco Meloni [2] and Cesare Miranda [3]

[1] Diabetes and Diabetic Foot Treatment Center, ASUGI Monfalcone Hospital, 34074 Monfalcone, Italy; andrea.michelli@asugi.sanita.fvg.it (A.M.); barbara.brunato@asugi.sanita.fvg.it (B.B.); enrica.barro@asugi.sanita.fvg.it (E.B.)
[2] Systems Medicine Department, Polyclinic Tor Vergata, Tor Vergata University, 00133 Rome, Italy
[3] Clinic of Endocrinology and Metabolism Diseases ASFO Pordenone Hospital, 33170 Pordenone, Italy
* Correspondence: roberto.daros@asugi.sanita.fvg.it

Abstract: Diabetic foot is a common complication of diabetes that affects quality and prognosis of life for patients and often requires hospitalization. Infection, alone or in association with ischemia, is the main cause of hospital admission and impacts prognosis. The aim of this study is to analyze the costs of diabetic foot lesions and assess factors that influence the economic impact, focusing on infection. We included all people with diabetes with a first visit for diabetic foot during 2018 in our diabetic foot center. Database interrogation identified 422 patients. Diabetic foot treatment required hospitalization for 242 patients (58%), while 180 (42%) were treated in outpatient services. Healing time was different between the two groups: it was 136 ± 124 days (mean ± SD) for outpatients and 194 ± 190 days for patients that require hospitalization ($p < 0.001$). Costs: Treatment of 422 patients for diabetic foot globally costs 2063 million EUR and the mean cost for patients is 4888 EUR, with hospital stay having a high impact on this, accounting for 88% of the costs. Infection impacts hospitalization duration and ischemia impacts healing time. Ischemia and infection prolonged hospitalization duration and costs. Our work underlines that hospital treatment costs have a high impact on total costs.

Keywords: diabetic foot ulcer; infection; hospitalization; peripheral arterial disease costs

1. Introduction

Diabetes mellitus has become a critical pandemic. According to the International Diabetes Federation [1], approximately 700 million people will live with diabetes until the year 2045.

According to the Italian National Institute of Statistics [2], there are more than 3 million people living with a diagnosis of diabetes in Italy, 5.3% of the total Italian population, and approximately another 1 million people who do not know that they have the disease.

Diabetic foot disease is a frequent complication of diabetes, with a high impact on patients' quality of life, and diabetic foot ulcer (DFU) is the main cause of non-traumatic limb amputation, an event that impacts the life of the patient and their family.

Distal peripheral neuropathy and peripheral arterial disease (PAD) are the two complications of diabetes underlying the development of diabetic foot. The risk of developing a lesion increases with one or both of these complications, particularly if associated with foot deformities or if the foot has already had ulcerations or previous amputations [3,4]. Recent data have highlighted that the annual incidence of diabetic foot ulcers has increased to 2% of patients, and up to 34% of patients with type 2 diabetes develop DFU at least once in their lifetime [5].

According to the Global Burden of Disease study [6], it was estimated that in 2016, 131.0 million (1.77%) people worldwide had lower-limb complications, equal to 34% of the diabetic population, of which 105.6 million had neuropathy alone, 18.6 million had DFU, and 6.8 million had lower-extremity amputations. These conditions account for 16.8 million years lived with disability (YLD) (2.07% of all YLDs), including 12.9 million for neuropathy, 2.5 million for foot ulcers, and 1.6 million for amputations [6].

These prevalence data are exacerbated by another dramatic fact: the risk of recurrence after healing of the ulcer. Ulcer recurrence is very frequent, and literature data highlight a risk of ulcer recurrence of 40% in the first year and 65% or more after 3 years [5]. For this reason, a previous injury or amputation constitutes a very high-risk factor for ulceration and in these conditions, the patient must be monitored frequently, a structured therapeutic education program must be started and indications must be given for the use of therapeutic footwear.

Diabetic foot disease not only impacts patients' quality of life [7,8] but is associated with a negative prognosis with a high mortality rate. Several studies reported that the five-year mortality rate due to DFU was 30.5%, while the five-year mortality rate due to minor and major amputation was 46.2% and 56.6%, respectively [9–13]. Infection, alone or in association with ischemia, is the main cause of hospital admissions and impacts prognosis [5,10].

These data justify all efforts to avoid major amputations, an event that impacts both patients' quality of life and results in a negative prognosis. The high impact of diabetic foot disease has resulted in this pathology being placed in the top 10 medical conditions [14].

In addition to the clinical impact, the diabetic foot has high management costs. The analysis of the Eurodiale study [15] highlights that the estimated cost of the treatment of a DFU is approximately EUR 10,000. In the UK, the National Health Service (NHS) spends between GBP 837 and 962 million annually on the treatment of ulcers and amputations [16], while direct costs for diabetic foot disease in the US in 2017 alone reached 80 billion USD [9–17], almost equal to the attributable cost of cancer in 2015 [18]. The aim of this study is to analyze the costs of healed foot lesions in people with diabetes and assess factors that may influence the economic impact, specifically diabetic foot infection (DFI).

2. Materials and Methods

This is a retrospective cross-sectional study using the administrative databases of the Monfalcone Hospital as the source of information. This study was conducted in accordance with the Helsinki Declaration of 1964 and its later amendments. We used a general consent system that was signed by patients on first visit, in which they agreed to their clinical data being used for clinical research, epidemiology, disease study and training, with the aim of improving knowledge, treatment and prevention. This study was based on the analysis of anonymous health administrative databases for which ethical committee approval was not required in Italy. Subjects included in our study were those with diabetes and DFUs recorded in our database from January to December 2018. All patients were treated in a third-level center in the presence of a multidisciplinary team directed by diabetologists and composed of vascular surgeons, orthopedists, nurses specializing in wounds, specialists in infectious diseases, interventional radiologists and orthopedic shoe technicians.

All of them were treated according to the local protocol in line with the International Working Group on Diabetic Foot Guidance [19] and the Italian consensus for treatment of PAD in diabetes [20]. These protocols include surgical debridement wound dressings, treatment of infection PAD, off-loading via irremovable or removable knee-high and ankle-high casts, and education. Regarding the cost analysis, we analyzed total costs and costs for hospital and community treatment. We also grouped patients based on the presence or absence of PAD and/or infection (according to the wound classification system of the University of Texas [21]) and the need for hospital stay.

3. Cost

Financial aspects were evaluated according to two main health conditions: inpatient and outpatient care. Extra hospitalization costs included first medical visit, control visit, wound care and dressing change, temporary shoes for acute-phase off-loading, and definitive therapeutic shoes. To each parameter, we assigned the unit costs based on Health Care System (HCS) evaluation.

Hence, the unit cost of any procedure, drug or visit included the total cost, regardless of whether expenses were for the HCS, patient, insurance, etc. Indirect costs, loss of working activity, time spent on visits, inability, etc., were not evaluated. We calculated costs individually for each patient based on resource utilization.

Clinical medical evaluation. Each patient received a first visit and 1 or more control visits. Costs of first visit (46.5 **EUR**) and control (21.5 EUR) are calculated based on HCS reimbursement.

Medications and topical treatment. The costs of medications (5 **EUR**) for topical treatment were calculated with HCS reimbursement independently of the setting for use of medications, i.e., home or hospital, and of the kind of dressing/therapy used.

Off-loading: Off-loading costs were calculated considering the total number of footwears, insoles, orthoses and casts prescribed for a patient and the unit cost of each type of off-loading. We maintain separate off-loading in the acute and chronic phases (Table 1).

Table 1. Summary of costs involved.

Acute-Phase Orthosis	Cost EUR	Chronic-Phase Definitive Orthosis	
Medical shoe	70	Preformed shoe	300
Brace	150	Brace	1800
Half cast	14	Prothesis	4000
Shoe + half cast	84	Custom made	900

Hospitalization cost was based on the diagnosis-related group (DRG) on hospitalization. Diagnoses recorded in hospital discharge records and specified in the International Classification of Diseases, 9th Revision [22], were examined and analyzed.

Hospital discharges with DRG (24th version) codes 213, 217, 218, 225, 226, 227, 233, 238, 263 and 264 were considered in the case of DFU.

The use of this parameter enabled easy comparison of costs (Table 2).

Table 2. Comparison of costs oh hospital discharges.

DRG	Description	Cost (EUR)	Occurrence	Cost Day Surgery (EUR/day)	Occurrence
113	Amputation for circulatory disease	13145	1		
213	Amputation for bone disease	8141	16		
217	Debridement and graft	11334	40	495	8
218	Surgical procedure on legs	7858	3		
225	Surgical procedure on foot	3164	12	3164	5
226	Surgical procedure on soft tissue with complications	6364	174	495	47
227	Surgical procedure on soft tissue without complications	1809	3	1809	2
233	Other procedures on bone/soft Tissue	9709	7		

Table 2. Cont.

DRG	Description	Cost (EUR)	Occurrence	Cost Day Surgery (EUR/day)	Occurrence
238	Osteomyelitis	5714	4		
263	Skin graft with complications	9690	10	453	1
264	Skin graft without Complications	5714	37	453	11
270	Other procedures on skin	1725	12		
Others			12		

Statistical analysis and cost calculations were performed using the SPSS statistical package, version 12.0.2 (SPSS, Chicago, IL, USA). Continuous variables are described as the mean and SD, whereas categorical variables are reported as the percentage.

4. Results

Of the 445 patients recruited, 23 were patients on secondary prevention without an active wound and thus excluded from this study. The remaining 422 patients were included and examined—127 (30%) were women, and 10 (2%) patients had type 1 diabetes while the remaining 412 (98%) had type 2 diabetes. The main baseline characteristics of the whole population are described in Table 3—a long history of diabetes, quite good metabolic control, obesity, and a high level of creatinine.

Table 3. Clinical characteristics of the whole population and groups of inpatients and outpatients.

Parameter	Total Population (n = 422) Mean ± SD	Hospitalized (n = 242 (57%)) Mean ± SD	Not hospitalized (n = 180 (43%)) Mean ± SD	p
Age (years)	72 ± 11	71 ± 12	74 ± 11	$p < 0.01$
Female n. (%)	127 (30%)	70 (29%)	57 (32%)	n.s.
BMI (m/kg^2)	27 ± 6	26 ± 6	28 ± 7	n.s.
Years of diabetes	19 ± 12	20 ± 11	18 ± 12	n.s.
HBA1c%	7.8 ± 2	8.1 ± 2	7.5 ± 1.5	n.s.
Creatinine (mg/dL)	1.96 ± 1.4	2.1 ± 1.5	1.56 ± 1.6	n.s.
Dialysis n.	16 (4%)	14 (6%)	2 (1%)	$p < 0.01$
CAD n.	178 (42%)	124 (51%)	54 (30%)	$p < 0.01$

CAD: Coronary Artery Disease. HbA1c: Glycated Haemoglobin. BMI: Body Max Index

The incidence of peripheral arterial disease with ischemia was very high. We found 213 people with this condition (50% of whole population), while infection was present in 121 patients (28% of the whole population).

We divided the population into two groups based on whether hospitalization was necessary: 57% required hospitalization, while 43% were managed on an outpatient basis. Hospitalization was required for peripheral ischemia and/or infection. All ischemic patients required hospitalization and 43% patients had infection. Hospitalized patients had a higher incidence of CAD, dialysis and were older. Control and history of diabetes, BMI, creatinine levels and sex were not associated with higher hospitalization rates.

Ulcer classification: Ulcer characteristics were completely different in the two groups. Inpatients presented with an ulcer of grade 3 Texas in 90% of cases—14% were 3A, 8% were 3B, 64% were 3C, and 14% were 3D. The remaining 10% presented ischemic lesions with grade 1 (74%) and 2 (26%). Outpatients did not show deep (grade 3) and/or ischemic ulcers (C), and lesions were classified as grades 1 (58%) and 2 (42%).

Among hospitalized patients, 242 patients accounted for 330 hospitalizations—191 for ischemia; 40 for ischemia and infection; 25 for infection without ischemia; 74 for surgical reconstruction, skin and dermal flap, and arthrodesis.

Clinical outcome: A total of 8 patients underwent major amputation while 38 patients underwent minor amputation (forefoot amputation). In 161 patients, surgical removal of metatarsal infected bone was performed, and 39 surgical procedures were limited to fingers.

The difference in the severity of the lesions between hospitalized and non-hospitalized patients also significantly affected the difference in the recovery time between the two groups—the recovery time was 136 ± 124 days (mean $\pm$ DS) for outpatients, and 194 ± 190 days for patients requiring hospitalization ($p < 0.001$).

The hospitalization rate resulted in a 1.37 hospitalization/patient ratio. While 25 were readmissions, new hospitalizations within 30 days of discharge from an acute care hospital accounted for 10% of the rate. The total cost of diabetic foot treatment of 422 patients was 2063 EUR, with the hospitalization cost of 1811 EUR accounting for 88%. We separately analyzed and compared patients treated only in the outpatient setting and patients managed in the hospital setting. For the 180 patients treated only in outpatient services, a first visit, a mean of 2 control visits, 47 for dressing applications, 1 for acute-phase orthosis and 1 chronic-phase orthosis were recorded. The individual extra hospitalization cost was 579 ± 293 EUR. The outpatient service costs of patients that also needed hospitalization were higher, as they required more control visits and higher costs for acute- and chronic-phase orthosis, with a total cost of 818 ± 603 EUR, as shown in Table 4.

Table 4. Outpatient service related costs.

Parameter	Patients Treated Only In Outpatient Services (n = 180)		Patients Treated in In- and Outpatient Services (n = 242)		Test T
	Mean $\pm$ DS	Cost (EUR) $\pm$ SD	Mean $\pm$ SD	Cost (EUR) $\pm$ SD	
First visit	1 ± 0	$46,5 \pm 0$	1 ± 0	$46,5 \pm 0$	n.s.
Control visits	2 ± 3	42 ± 59	4 ± 3.7	82 ± 80	<0.01
Dressing	47 ± 37	235 ± 184	48 ± 40	238 ± 200	n.s
Acute phase Orthosis	1 ± 0	44 ± 39	1 ± 0	70 ± 67	<0.01
Chronic phase Orthosis	1 ± 0	212 ± 207	1 ± 0	372 ± 517	<0.01
Total		579 ± 293		811 ± 603	<0.01

The 330 hospitalizations were divided into 256 ordinary hospitalizations and 74 day surgery appointments. The mean duration of hospital stay was 10 ± 10 days (mean $\pm$ SD), and the mean cost was 6855 ± 2393 euros (mean $\pm$ SD). The mean duration of day surgery was 1 day, and the mean cost was 761 ± 764 euros (mean $\pm$ SD). Hospitalization analysis based on clinical characteristics causative of hospitalization such as ischemia and infection highlights that DFI impacts hospitalization length, while ischemia impacts healing time—together, ischemia and infection prolong hospitalization duration and costs (Table 5).

In our group, eight patients underwent major amputation, and the DRG cost of major amputation in vascular patients was 11,127 EUR. The total costs for these patients were not analyzed because they were treated through another surgical service at our hospital.

Table 5. Hospital stay, healing time and hospitalization costs.

Parameter	No Ischemia Infection (n = 25)	Ischemia Not Infection (n = 191)	Ischemia and Infection (n = 40)	Test T Ischemia With/Without Infection	Test T Infection With/Without Ischemia
Hospital stay (days), mean ± DS	12.5 ± 9.7	9 ± 9	16 ± 13	< 0.01	n.s
Healing time (days), mean ± SD	135 ± 121	263 ± 243	268 ± 287	n.s.	0.04
Hospitalization costs (EUR) ± DS	6486 ± 2860	6514 ± 2632	7657 ± 2175	0.01	n.s.

5. Discussion

This study highlights a year of activity involving the diabetic foot at a reference center, and presents a large series of cases—422 cases included. Data show that a high percentage of patients (57%) have complicated injuries that require treatment in hospital. Furthermore, in addition to having serious injuries, these patients are more fragile—they are older with the ischemic heart disease and dialysis. These conditions impact prognosis and recovery times, which are significantly longer than for patients treated on an outpatient basis. The cost analysis also highlights a great impact of this complication from an economic point of view. Hospitalization accounts for most of the costs in the management of diabetic foot syndrome, 88% of the total cost. Ischemia and infection, combined or alone, are the causes of hospitalization—they impact the duration of hospital stay, healing time and costs.

This is the first economic evaluation of diabetic foot care at Monfalcone Hospital. The present study, carried out at a third-level center with a multidisciplinary team, highlights that dedicated care for diabetic foot has better clinical outcomes and lower costs compared to standard treatments. The clinical advantage of optimal care can be clearly seen through the reduction in the frequency of foot complications or negative evolution such as amputation. In fact, DFD causes an increase in morbidity and frequent hospital admissions, worsening recovery times and the possibility of particularly disabling sequelae, such as amputation of the lower limbs.

Diabetes represents a pathology with high treatment costs—approximately 11 billion—per year for the Italian National Health Service [23], accounting 10% of the annual budget (111 billion euros in 2018) [24]. The study based on the ARNO Diabetes Observatory analyzed the average cost of healthcare for diabetic patients in 2018—the average cost for each patient was 2833 euros and the greatest impact on overall costs was the cost of hospitalization, which represented 40% of the total costs (1152 euros) [23]. As regards specific analyses on the costs of diabetic foot, a recent study, conducted in Tuscany, evaluated healthcare costs for a large population cohort [25]. Of the 730 patients who developed a DFU in the period 2015–2018, the analysis found that 114 had an amputation (15.6%) with an annual per capita cost calculated at EUR 12,146, compared to a patient without amputation and a cost of EUR 7864 [25].

The burden of diabetes is represented in particular by hospital admissions. Diabetic foot is one of the most expensive complications of diabetes and can be a major economic and public health burden. Wound resolution is not an immediate target and data from this study, with a mean healing time longer than 5 months, confirm the important impact on public health as well as underlining the efforts to obtain wound resolution.

Considering that the hospitalization cost is the main cost in the treatment of diabetic foot, efforts must be made to optimize hospitalization times and management of the hospitalized patient. To achieve this, in our center, we use a multidisciplinary approach dedicated to diabetic foot, with close coordination between specialists to optimize patient treatment and reduce the duration of hospital stay. The average length of hospital stay was

10 days and the average cost of each hospitalization was less than EUR 7000, confirming the effectiveness of this approach compared to approaches presented in other studies [26–28].

The readmission rate, i.e., new hospitalizations within 30 days of discharge from an acute hospital, represents a qualitative index that can be used to evaluate the approach to diabetic foot lesions. A treatment with frequent re-admissions is not clinically effective not cost-effective. The readmission rate obtained in this study was 10%, which is relatively low compared to the readmission rate reported in the literature, higher than 20–30% [29]. Reasons for this outcome include complete resolution of ischemia and infection before hospital discharge including acute surgical treatment of infection and definitive surgical treatment as well as the combination of revascularization and subsequent surgical treatment of the foot.

In one year, the expenditure for 422 patients suffering from diabetic foot was 2 million euros, with a significant impact of hospitalization (87%) on the total cost, confirming the literature data. Hospitalization was necessary in 58% of patients, a very high percentage that can be explained by the fact that our third-level center receives the most complex cases, which most frequently require hospitalization. Furthermore, by analyzing the hospitalized patients, we found a high incidence of vascular and cardiovascular diseases (90%), so we included more fragile patients requiring hospitalization.

Our analysis then evaluated the factors influencing the cost of hospitalization by evaluating the impact of infection, ischemia or both conditions. The more complicated patients, who presented a combination of ischemia and infection, had significantly higher hospitalization costs. Likewise, the length of hospitalization for these patients was significantly longer. Analyzing the clinical effects of infection and ischemia by evaluating them individually, it appears that infection significantly increases the duration of hospitalization while ischemia negatively affects recovery time. Thus, ischemic patients have significantly longer recovery times. These data can be used for preventive treatment. In particular, the data indicate the importance of preventing infectious evolution in patients with diabetic foot lesions, especially if they are also ischemic. Avoiding infection could have a huge impact on saving the foot and treatment costs.

An American study, based on data from medical and pharmaceutical claims from 2000 and 2001, included outpatients and inpatients with or without peripheral arterial disease. The results of the work showed an average cost per lesion of 13,179 USD (approximately EUR 10,914), ranging from 5218 USD (4321 EUR) for patients without PAD compared to 23,372 USD (19,357 EUR) for patients with PAD [30]. In our work, we did not find this high difference between vascular and non-vascular patients, as PAD had a significant impact on recovery times but not on costs. The possible explanation for our results is the usually chronic and not acute ischemia, therefore enabling planning hospitalization without resorting to urgent hospitalization. Planned hospitalization with short revascularization and surgical treatment times enables a reduction in hospitalization times and, therefore, a relative reduction in costs.

On the other hand, higher costs were involved for the treatment of patients with PAD and infection. The increase in costs in these cases is justified not only by the need for hospitalization, with higher rates of hospitalization, but also by the use of antibiotics, the need for amputation, revascularization, the need for multiple surgical interventions and the duration of hospitalization.

As the data in our work show, outpatient services account for approximately 8% of the total costs. The largest outpatient service costs relate to preventive footwear provided to the patient. This is a device used to prevent relapses, given the high rate reported in the literature. We also know that a new injury has a decidedly significant impact on quality of life and costs. It therefore becomes essential to educate the patient, who is at high risk of ulceration having already had a lesion, on the correct use of these devices. Reducing ulcer recurrence represents a challenge in the treatment of diabetic foot.

6. Limitations

We must also analyze the limits of our work. In this study, we included a white European population without racial/ethnic diversity, which raises concerns regarding the generalizability of our findings to other ethnic groups. Consequently, our results would benefit from verification in diverse populations. The use of data from an administrative database may present coding errors, so we integrated administrative data with clinical data to minimize the occurrence of missing data. In any case, it is possible that some of the diagnoses of foot ulceration identified by the ICD-9 (International Classification of Disease, 9th Revision) codes are not entirely representative of the pathological state of interest. The direct costs were calculated on the basis of the 2018 reimbursement rates, which remained unchanged in Italy but could be different from current costs in other countries. Finally, our analysis only concerns direct costs, as we have not calculated indirect costs, which include sickness absence, loss of production, temporary disability and early retirement. A systematic review [31] reported that indirect costs for diabetic foot ulcers in Europe range from USD 1027 [15] to 1476 [32], and those for amputations range from USD 1043 [15] to 1442 [32], while indirect costs per ulcer with infection were not available.

The clinical outcome could be influenced by other factors not evaluated in this study, for example patient compliance, but this is a one-year real-life study with a large cohort and prospective monitoring aimed at evaluating clinical practice daily without predetermined intervention options.

7. Conclusions

This study confirms the complexity of the treatment of diabetic foot, with the need for inpatient and outpatient treatments with long times to achieve healing of the lesions. This study also highlights the need for a multidisciplinary approach to optimize treatment times and patient outcomes [33].

This complexity is confirmed by the high costs. In particular, our analysis confirmed that hospital treatment has a significant impact on the costs of diabetic foot treatment. These data provide reference points in the analysis of diabetic foot treatment.

We have highlighted that clinical conditions such as ischemia and infection are increasingly responsible for hospitalizations, influence the duration of hospitalization and impact the outcome. We believe that strategies aimed at avoiding delays in patient referral are able to reduce the impact on costs and improve clinical outcome, especially if combined with timely institution of antibiotic therapy and early vascular intervention. The goal must be to prevent limb loss.

The presence of multidisciplinary diabetic foot centers can reduce disease progression and amputation [34]. In these centers, there should be limb salvage teams that deal with prevention, as the surveillance and management of foot ulcers through a multidisciplinary approach can improve outcomes [35,36].

Our data suggest that among the various competing factors, infection affects the need for hospitalization, also increasing the economic health burden associated with the treatment of diabetic foot ulcers. Efforts should therefore be made to avoid this impactful event. Further research and multicenter prospective studies are recommended to identify more variables that influence cost management.

In conclusion, the present study clearly suggests that an optimal multidisciplinary approach can limit costs for the treatment of DFUs. A preventive approach with a reduction in infections and rapid referral to reference centers could also be even more effective in reducing the clinical and economic impacts of diabetic foot.

Author Contributions: Conceptualization, R.D.R. and C.M.; methodology, C.M.; software, R.D.R.; validation, R.A., B.B. and E.B; formal analysis, A.M.; investigation, R.A.; resources, R.D.R.; data curation, R.D.R.; writing—original draft preparation, R.D.R.; writing—review and editing, M.M.; visualization, E.B.; supervision, M.M.; project administration, R.D.R. All authors have read and agreed to the published version of the manuscript.

Funding: This research received no external funding.

Institutional Review Board Statement: This study was conducted in accordance with the Helsinki Declaration of 1964 and its later amendments. According to the Italian Medicines Agency det. 20/03/2008 on retrospective observational studies on anonymous data, preemptive approval by an ethics committee was not mandatory and given that the study collected anonymous data, not referable to specific individuals, approval by one or more ethical committee(s) was not requested.

Informed Consent Statement: We used a general consent system that was signed by patients on first visit, in which they agreed to their clinical data being used for clinical research, epidemiology, disease study and training.

Data Availability Statement: The original contributions presented in the study are included in the article, further inquiries can be directed to the corresponding author/s.

Conflicts of Interest: The authors declare no conflict of interest.

References

1. International Diabetes Federation. IDF Diabetes Atlas, Nine Edition 2019. Available online: http://www.diabetesatlas.org (accessed on 15 July 2020).
2. ISTAT 2017. Available online: http://www.epicentro.iss.it/igea.it/ (accessed on 13 October 2021).
3. Boulton, A.J.; Armstrong, D.G. American Diabetes Association; American Association of Clinical Endocrinologists. Comprehensive foot examination and risk assessment: A report of the task force of the foot care interest group of the American Diabetes Association, with endorsement by the American Association of Clinical Endocrinologists. *Diabetes Care* **2008**, *31*, 1679–1685. [PubMed]
4. van Netten, J.J.; Price, P.E.; International Working Group on the Diabetic Foot. Prevention of foot ulcers in the at-risk patient with diabetes: A systematic review. *Diabetes Metab. Res. Rev.* **2016**, *32*, 84–98. [CrossRef]
5. Armstrong, D.G.; Boulton, A.J.M. Diabetic Foot Ulcers and Their Recurrence. *N. Engl. J. Med.* **2017**, *15*, 2367–2375. [CrossRef] [PubMed]
6. Zhang, Y.; Lazzarini, P.A. Global disability burdens of diabetes-related lower-extremity complications in 1990 and 2016. *Diabetes Care* **2020**, *43*, 964–974. [CrossRef] [PubMed]
7. Boulton, A.J.; Vileikyte, L.; Ragnarson-Tennvall, G.; Apelqvist, J. The global burden of diabetic foot disease. *Lancet* **2005**, *366*, 1719–1724. [CrossRef] [PubMed]
8. Jeffcoate, W.J.; Price, P.E. Randomised controlled trial of the use of three dressing preparations in the management of chronic ulceration of the foot in diabetes. *Health Technol. Assess* **2009**, *54*, 1–86. [CrossRef] [PubMed]
9. Armstrong, D.G.; Swerdlow, M.A. Five year mortality and direct costs of care for people with diabetic foot complications are comparable to cancer. *J. Foot Ankle Res.* **2020**, *13*, 2–5. [CrossRef]
10. Huang, Y.-Y.; Lin, C.-W. Survival and associated risk factors in patients with diabetes and amputations caused by infectious foot gangrene. *J. Foot Ankle Res.* **2018**, *11*, 1. [CrossRef] [PubMed]
11. Walsh, J.W.; Hoffstad, O.J. Association of diabetic foot ulcer and death in a population-based cohort from the United Kingdom. *Diabet Med.* **2016**, *33*, 1491–1498. [CrossRef] [PubMed]
12. Morbach, S.; Furchert, H. Long-term prognosis of diabetic foot patients and their limbs: Amputation and death over the course of a decade. *Diabetes Care* **2012**, *35*, 2021–2027. [CrossRef] [PubMed]
13. Lavery, L.A.; Hunt, N.A. Impact of chronic kidney disease on survival after amputation in individuals with diabetes. *Diabetes Care* **2010**, *33*, 2365–2369. [CrossRef] [PubMed]
14. Lazzarini, P.A.; Pacella, R.E. Diabetes-related lower-extremity complications are a leading cause of the global burden of disability. *Diabet Med.* **2018**, *35*, 1297–1299. [CrossRef] [PubMed]
15. Prompers, L.; Huijberts, M. Resource utilisation and costs associated with the treatment of diabetic foot ulcers. Prospective data from the Eurodiale Study. *Diabetologia* **2008**, *51*, 1826–1834. [CrossRef] [PubMed]
16. American Diabetes Association. Economic Costs of Diabetes in the U.S. in 2017. *Diabetes Care* **2018**, *41*, 917–928. [CrossRef] [PubMed]
17. Kerr, M.; Barron, E. The cost of diabetic foot ulcers and amputations to the National Health Service in England. *Diabet Med.* **2019**, *36*, 995–1002. [CrossRef] [PubMed]
18. Economic Impact of Cancer. Available online: https://www.cancer.org/cancer/cancer-basics/economic-impact-of-cancer.html (accessed on 19 October 2021).
19. Schaper, N.C.; Van Netten, J.J.; International Working Group on the Diabetic Foot (IWGDF). Prevention and management of foot problems in diabetes: A Summary Guidance for Daily Practice 2015, based on the IWGDF guidance documents. *Diabetes Res. Clin. Pract.* **2017**, *124*, 84–92. [CrossRef] [PubMed]
20. Aiello, A.; Anichini, R.; Italian Society of Diabetes; Italian Society of Radiology; Italian Society of Vascular Endovascular Surgery. Treatment of peripheral arterial disease in diabetes: A consensus of the Italian Societies of Diabetes (SID, AMD), Radiology (SIRM) and Vascular Endovascular Surgery (SICVE). *Nutr. Metab. Cardiovasc. Dis.* **2014**, *24*, 355–369. [CrossRef] [PubMed]

21. Armstrong, D.G.; Lavery, L.A. Validation of a diabetic wound classification system. The contribution of depth, infection, and ischemia to risk of amputation. *Diabetes Care* **1998**, *21*, 855–859. [CrossRef] [PubMed]
22. ICD-9-CM. International Classification of Diseases, 9th revision. 2002. Available online: http://wwwsalute.gov.it (accessed on 15 December 2021).
23. Bonora, E.; Cataudella, S. Under the mandate of the Italian Diabetes Society. Clinical burden of diabetes in Italy in 2018: A look at a systemic disease from the ARNO Diabetes Observatory. *BMJ Open Diabetes Res. Care* **2020**, *8*, e001291. [CrossRef] [PubMed]
24. Gazzetta Ufficiale della Repubblica Italiana. Ripartizione del Fondo Sanitario Nazionale. Available online: http://www.regioni.it/news/2019/02/28/riparto-fondo-sanitario-nazionale-2018-delibera-cipe-28-11-2018-gazzetta-ufficiale-n-49-del-27-febbraio-2019-595365 (accessed on 1 October 2023).
25. Seghieri, C.; Ferrè, F. Healthcare costs of diabetic foot disease in Italy: Estimates for event and state costs. *Eur. J. Health Econ.* **2022**, *24*, 167–169. [CrossRef] [PubMed]
26. Nieto-Gil, P.; Ortega-Avila, A.B. Hospitalisation Cost of Patients with Diabetic Foot Ulcers in Valencia (Spain) in the Period 2009–2013: A Retrospective Descriptive Analysis. *Int. J. Environ. Res. Public Health* **2018**, *24*, 1831. [CrossRef]
27. Hicks, C.W.; Selvarajah, S. Burden of Infected Diabetic Foot Ulcers on Hospital Admissions and Costs. *Ann. Vasc. Surg.* **2016**, *33*, 149–158. [CrossRef] [PubMed]
28. Lu, Q.; Wang, J. Cost of Diabetic Foot Ulcer Management in China: A 7-Year Single-Center Retrospective Review. *Diabetes Metab. Syndr. Obes.* **2020**, *13*, 4249–4260. [CrossRef] [PubMed]
29. King, K.R.; Hatch, D.C., Jr. A Critical Look At Readmissions For Patients With Diabetic Foot Infections. *Podiatry Today* **2018**, *31*, 12–16.
30. Stockl, K.; Vanderplas, A. Costs of lower-extremity ulcers among patients with diabetes. *Diabetes Care* **2004**, *27*, 2129–2134. [CrossRef] [PubMed]
31. Tchero, H.; Kangambega, P. Cost of diabetic foot in France, Spain, Italy, Germany and United Kingdom: A systematic review. *Ann. Endocrinol.* **2018**, *79*, 67–74. [CrossRef] [PubMed]
32. Happich, M.; John, J.; Stamenitis, S.; Clouth, J.; Polnau, D. The quality of life and economic burden of neuropathy in diabetic patients in Germany in 2002-results from the diabetic microvascular complications (DIMICO) study. *Diabetes Res. Clin. Pract.* **2008**, *81*, 223–230. [CrossRef] [PubMed]
33. Meloni, M.; Giurato, L. Effect of a multidisciplinary team approach in patients with diabetic foot ulcers on major adverse limb events (MALEs): Systematic review and meta-analysis for the development of the Italian guidelines for the treatment of diabetic foot syndrome. *Acta Diabetol.* **2024**, *24*, 2246–2249. [CrossRef] [PubMed]
34. Williams, D.T.; Majeed, M.U. A diabetic foot service established by a department of vascular surgery: An observational study. *Ann. Vasc. Surg.* **2012**, *26*, 700–706. [CrossRef] [PubMed]
35. Zayed, H.; Halawa, M. Improving limb salvage rate in diabetic patients with critical leg ischaemia using a multidisciplinary approach. *Int. J. Clin. Pract.* **2009**, *63*, 855–858. [CrossRef]
36. Driver, V.R.; Goodman, R.A. The impact of a podiatric lead limb preservation team on disease outcomes and risk prediction in the diabetic lower extremity: A retrospective cohort study. *J. Am. Podiatr. Med. Assoc.* **2010**, *100*, 235–241.

Disclaimer/Publisher's Note: The statements, opinions and data contained in all publications are solely those of the individual author(s) and contributor(s) and not of MDPI and/or the editor(s). MDPI and/or the editor(s) disclaim responsibility for any injury to people or property resulting from any ideas, methods, instructions or products referred to in the content.

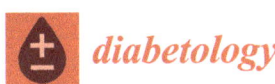 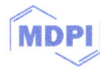

Article

Utility of Flash Glucose Monitoring to Determine Glucose Variation Induced by Different Doughs in Persons with Type 2 Diabetes

Maria Antonietta Taras [1], Sara Cherchi [1], Ilaria Campesi [2], Valentina Margarita [2], Gavino Carboni [2], Paola Rappelli [2,3] and Giancarlo Tonolo [1,*]

[1] Diabetology Operative Unit, After Asl Gallura.P.O. San Giovanni di Dio Via a. Moro, 07026 Olbia, Italy; anto.ta@inwind.it (M.A.T.)
[2] Department of Biomedical Sciences, University of Sassari, 07100 Sassari, Italy; icampesi@uniss.it (I.C.); vmargarita@uniss.it (V.M.); rappelli@uniss.it (P.R.)
[3] Mediterranean Center for Disease Control, 07100 Sassari, Italy
* Correspondence: giancarlo.tonolo@aslgallura.it

Citation: Taras, M.A.; Cherchi, S.; Campesi, I.; Margarita, V.; Carboni, G.; Rappelli, P.; Tonolo, G. Utility of Flash Glucose Monitoring to Determine Glucose Variation Induced by Different Doughs in Persons with Type 2 Diabetes. *Diabetology* 2024, 5, 129–140. https://doi.org/10.3390/diabetology5010010

Academic Editor: Bernd Stratmann

Received: 12 January 2024
Revised: 1 March 2024
Accepted: 7 March 2024
Published: 12 March 2024

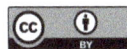

Copyright: © 2024 by the authors. Licensee MDPI, Basel, Switzerland. This article is an open access article distributed under the terms and conditions of the Creative Commons Attribution (CC BY) license (https://creativecommons.org/licenses/by/4.0/).

Abstract: (1) Background: It has been previously shown that sourdough bread, compared to commercial yeast bread, elicits a lower postprandial glycemic and insulinemic response in patients with impaired glucose tolerance (IGT). Aims: Our aim was to evaluate the following aspects in persons with type 2 diabetes (T2DM): (1) glucose variations induced by three different doughs: X = bread prepared with functional alkaline biocrystal water, Y = sourdough-leavened bread, and W = bakery yeast bread; (2) the utility of flash glucose monitoring (FGM) to measure GL. (2) Methods: Twelve T2DM following diets (six males, diabetes duration 10.9 ± 1.3 years with no complications, Hba1c < 7.0%), after 12 h of fasting, consumed 180 g of the study breads leavened/matured for 48 (X), 8 (Y), and 4 h (W) at room temperature with 200 mL of water, in a random order, in single-blind conditions, on three different days. All patients had FGM running for the entire period of the experiments. Insulin was determined by capillary blood obtained for the basal and peak glucose concentrations. (3) Results: The peak glucose and peak insulin concentrations were significantly ($p < 0.05$) higher for W versus both X and Y, without significant differences between X and Y. The area under the curve of glucose variations for over 240 min was significantly higher in W than X ($p < 0.01$) and Y ($p < 0.05$), without significant differences between X and Y. (4) Conclusions: (1) Bread prepared with biocrystal water has the same lower GL of sourdough bread compared to bakery yeast bread, and it is easier to manage its leavening/maturation period; (2) FGM is a reliable method for determining rapid glucose changes in response to a carbohydrate meal in persons with type 2 diabetes.

Keywords: glucose index; biocrystal water; sourdough bread; interstitial glucose monitoring; type 2 diabetes mellitus

1. Introduction

Bread is one of the most relevant sources of carbohydrates, not only in the Mediterranean diet. Bread has a high glycemic index (GI) [1,2], inducing a faster exposure to glucose over time, but it is the actual content of carbohydrates that drives a longer exposure to glucose, the so-called glucose load (GL). In other words, the GI is a ranking of how quickly a food raises blood sugar, while the GL takes into account the GI and the amount of carbohydrate in a serving. The GL is then a measure of the total impact of that kind of food on blood sugar levels, and it is calculated by multiplying the GI by the amount of carbohydrate in a serving, as clearly indicated by different online calculators such as www.omnicalculator.com/health/glycemic-load (accessed on 10 July 2020). An example is given by watermelon, which has a GI of 79 (moderately high), but, in a normal serving, the GL is only 4, since it is mostly water. A reduction in the GL is considered favorable to health in diabetic or pre-diabetic persons in which a high GL is responsible for a greater and longer increase in postprandial glycemia associated with cardiovascular disease [3–6]. In non-diabetic subjects, high-GL food may be associated with cancer [7] or with Nonalcoholic Fatty Liver Disease [8], particularly in the presence of insulin resistance. The possible beneficial effects obtained in long-term interventions in which low-GL food is administered are highlighted by the decrease in fasting insulin and pro-inflammatory markers such as C-reactive protein, which are proven to be linked with obesity-associated diseases [9]. Several studies have shown that the sourdough fermentation of wheat flour dough significantly decreases the glucose load of bread, since the starch has a reduced amount of glucose [10–12]. In addition to the sourdough fermentation of wheat flour, to date, different strategies to reduce the GL of bread have been evaluated, but the preparation of most of these breads is very difficult and not applicable in real life, reducing the possibility of preparing bread with a low GL for the entire population. Preparing bread with low salt content has become a nearly-zero-cost intervention directed toward the whole population; it can reduce salt intake and reduce the spread of hypertension and cardiovascular risk in the population [13]. In the same direction, the adoption of a low-GL bread by the entire population might be also an additional strategy for a significant reduction in cardiovascular disease in the population. This goal is achievable if the bread can be prepared with timeliness and costs favorable to bakers.

Continuous subcutaneous glucose monitoring (CGM) is now widely accepted as an alternative means to conventional finger-prick tests for measuring glucose levels in individuals with diabetes mellitus, particularly those who utilize intensive insulin treatment [14–16]. Flash glucose monitoring (FGM) is a wireless method that uses a sensor to monitor interstitial fluid glucose functioning as a hybrid between blood glucose measurement with a glucometer (SMBG) and CGM. Patients can obtain near-real-time glucose levels without finger pricks by regularly scanning the sensor. FGM has been proven to be an economical alternative to CGM [17,18]. More than 99.9% of the interstitial glucose measurements by FGM and capillary glucose pairs are within the combined zones of A and B of the consensus and Clarke error grids [19,20].

Recently, we become aware of a particular kind of bread with a long maturation/fermentation time (between 24 and 48 h) at room temperature, the dough of which is prepared with functional alkaline (biocrystal) water at pH 9.0, which has glucose/fructose content some 10 times lower than usual bread.

In the light of these considerations, the two aims of this work were as follows:
(1) To compare the GL of the dough prepared with functional alkaline (biocrystal) water (X) against one prepared with "mother" yeast, sourdough-leavened bread (Y), and one prepared with a commercial rapid leavening dough, bakery yeast bread (W), in persons with type 2 diabetes (T2DM);
(2) To investigate the utility of FGM to measure rapid glucose changes after a GL in T2DM.

2. Patients and Methods

This work has been carried out in accordance with The Code of Ethics of the World Medical Association [1964 Declaration of Helsinki and its later amendments] for experiments involving humans. The study was approved by the local Ethics Committee on 14 July 2020 (NP 248/2020/CE), and informed consent was obtained from each participant.

2.1. Patients

Twelve type 2 persons with diabetes (T2DM, Table 1) in good metabolic control without drug therapy, regularly attending our Diabetology Operative Unit, were enrolled in the study after informed consent was obtained. Female patients had been in physiological menopause for at least two years. Patients did not have evidence of celiac disease or gluten intolerance.

Table 1. Baseline anthropometric and biochemical data of the twelve T2DM.

Age [years]	69.9 ± 1.3	LDL Cholesterol [mmol/L]	2.91 ± 0.5
HbA1c [mol/L %]	49.8 ± 1.8 6.7 ± 0.25	Total Cholesterol [mmol/L]	4.92 ± 0.6
BMI	27.9 ± 1.2	Triglycerides [mmol/L]	1.42 ± 0.3
Diabetes duration [years]	10.9 ± 1.3	HDL Cholesterol [mmol/L]	1.44 ± 0.1
Systolic blood pressure [mmHg]	119 ± 3.1	SGOT [nkat/L]	415 ± 39
Diastolic blood pressure [mmHg]	75 ± 1.2	SGPT [nkat/L]	421 ± 49
Creatinine [μmol/L]	75.4 ± 4.1	γGT [nkat/L]	445 ± 69

Data are represented as mean SEM.

Patients were randomly offered 180 g of three different breads prepared in the form of "focaccia", cooked on the morning of the experiment, with 200 mL of still water at 08:00 a.m. after at least 10 h of fasting. The bread was consumed within 15 min, and during the test, participants remained seated quietly for the entire observation period of 240 min. All subjects followed a standard normal-caloric balanced diet (57% carbohydrates with <10% simple carbohydrates, 25% fat with <10% saturated fat, 18% protein, salt < 6 g per day, fibres 16 g/1000 Kcal) at least three weeks before starting the study and maintained it throughout the entire observation period. In detail, they ate the same dinner the evening before the entire observation period for the different tests. Patients were asked to maintain the same usual physical activity during the experimental period.

All patients had FGM running (FreeStyle Libre ® from Abbott, Chicago, IL, USA) from at least 24 h before the first test day and expiring at least 24 h after the third test day. Blood samples for serum insulin and blood glucose were collected basally and at the peak glucose concentration, as determined by FGM measurements being in stable phases. All subjects ate the different breads on three different occasions that were three/four days apart.

2.2. Study Breads

The three different types of bread with standardized compositions and fermentation/maturation times at room temperature are described in Table 2.

Table 2. Doughs' compositions.

	Flour [g]	Yeast [g]	Biocrystal Water [g]	Salt [g]	Extra Virgin Olive Oil [g]	Homemade Mother Yeast [g]	Tap Water [g]	Fermentation/Maturation [h]
X	1000	2	700	25	30	0	0	48
Y	1000	2	0	25	30	250	600	8
W	1000	2	0	25	30	0	700	4

Doughs' compositions. X = Functional alkaline water bread; Y = sourdough-leavened bread; W = bakery yeast bread. Doughs were prepared to finish fermentation maturation time together and cooked in the morning just before the experiments.

The biocrystal alkaline water used in this study was functional alkaline water, obtained through purification with ceramics with trace elements, antioxidants, ionization, and hydrogenation. Specifically, the water was initially micro-filtered through activated carbon and then, through a process of reverse osmosis, the pure osmotic water passed through a system of bioceramics and semi-precious metals (tourmaline, zeolite, hematite), becoming alkaline functional water at pH 9.0 (www.biocrystalacquaalcalina.com/acqua-biocrystal, accessed on 20 March 2021).

2.3. Isolation of Microbial Flora by Culture-Dependent Microbiological Analysis

To determine the presumptive lactic acid bacteria [LAB] in the three dough samples (X, Y, and W), 10 g of each dough was mixed with 40 mL of sterile NaCl solution (0.9% weight/volume) and homogenized in a classic blender. Tenfold dilution series for each suspension were made, and 100 μL of each dilution was plated in triplicate on de Man–Rogosa–Sharpe (MRS) agar medium (Biolife, Bellingham, WA, USA), supplemented with 10 mg/L of cycloheximide (Sigma-Aldrich, St. Louis, MO, USA, Merck, Rahway, NJ, USA) and in Luria Bertani (LB) agar (Sigma-Aldrich, Merck) medium. All plates were incubated at 30 °C for 48 h. The procedures were performed in triplicate. Up to 50 colonies were then randomly picked from the lowest countable dilutions and were grown in 5 mL of MRS broth (Biolife) at 30 °C for 24 h.

2.4. Bacterial Identification by MALDI-TOF Mass Spectrometry

Isolated bacteria were identified by MALDI-TOF mass spectrometry according to the "direct colony extraction technique" [21]. Briefly, a small portion of a single colony was directly smeared as a thin film onto a target plate (VITEK® MS-DS SLIDE, Biomerieux, Marcy-l'Étoile, France), using a 1 μL loop (performed in two spots for each strain), immediately followed by the addition of 1 μL of α-cyano-4-hydroxycinnamic acid (VITEK MS-CHCA, BioMerieux) for each sample spot. The samples were allowed to dry at room temperature before MS analysis [22]. To calibrate the mass spectrometer, the *E. coli* ATCC 8739 strain was inoculated on the central spot of the target slide, useful for every acquisition group. Matrix solution (α-cyano-4-hydroxycinnamic acid, BioMérieux) was also tested alone as a negative control. For the analysis, each spot was irradiated with 500 laser shots at 50 Hz, and spectra were acquired (mass range of 2 to 20 kDa in the linear model). Identification results were obtained by transferring the data from the Vitek acquisition station to the Vitek MS analysis server. Confidence values for each tested strain were calculated using the software MK2/2020. According to the manufacturer, values between 60.0 and 99.9 indicated the reliable discrimination of species or species groups [23].

2.5. Glucose and Insulin Determinations during the Study

During the three test days, participants performed manual scanning of the sensor every 5 min after eating to identify the peak glucose concentration. The analysis of the graph obtained during the 4-h study allowed the calculation of the area under the curve (AUC) of glucose variations after the bread was eaten (Figure 1).

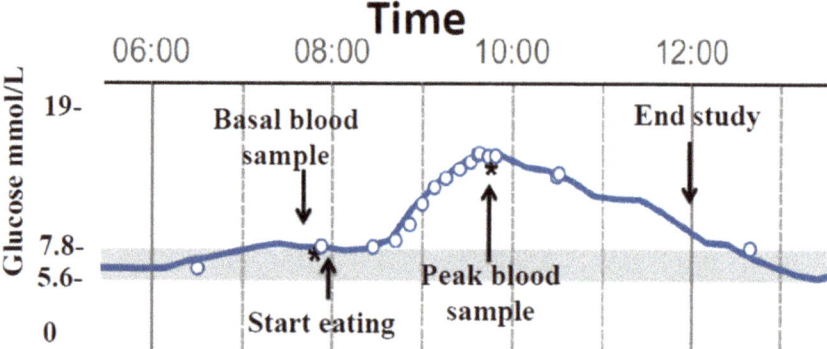

Figure 1. Representation of the interstitial glucose modifications during the one-day test in one T2DM. In the figure, the start eating = 08:00 a.m. and end study day = 12:00 a.m. times are indicated. * indicates blood sampling: at basal and at peak. ° indicates the moment of scanning the sensor; this was carried out frequently after having eaten the bread to identify the peak of glucose increase after the meal.

This was obtained with Excel using the trapezoidal formula, dividing the 240-min experiment into 5-min intervals. During the study, serum samples were collected by finger pricks for blood glucose and insulin determination at the basal concentration, before eating the bread, and at the peak blood glucose concentration, as determined by the "flat" position of the arrow in the FGM display. The first blood drop from the finger prick was used to determine blood glucose (blood glucose readings were performed on the built-in meter free style® glucometer, Abbott, used to scan interstitial glucose variations over time), while an additional 8–10 drops were collected in a conical 1.0 mL Eppendorf vial and centrifuged for 20 min at 4000 rpm with a refrigerated Eppendorf centrifuge, 5427R, and the supernatant was stored at $-20\ °C$ until it was assayed for insulin determination. Insulin was determined in all twelve T2DM for the three different test days in the same assay using a sandwich immunological test based on the principle of chemiluminescence (LIAISON Insulin kit; DiaSorin, Saluggia, Italy). Briefly, 100 µL of serum was diluted with 210 µL of the LIASON Endocrinology Diluent buffer, and after being mixed well, 150 µL of the mixture was used to determine insulin concentrations. All samples were assayed in duplicate. The assay was not affected by hemoglobin values up to 1000 mg/dL, and the analytical sensitivity was 0.5 µIU/mL. The evaluation of serum insulin response along with the glycemic one is more effective in characterizing glucose metabolism impairment [24,25].

2.6. Statistical Analysis

The sample size was calculated based on preliminary data and considering a minimum power of 80% (type-II error, 1-beta), 5% of significance (alpha: 0.05), and a medium effect size (f = 0.25), using Gpower software(GH/2021). Descriptive summary statistics for continuous data numbers, means, and standard errors of the mean (SEMs) were performed for all measurements. Multiple linear regression analysis was used to determine the predictors of significance at the determined points (from 0 to 240 min at 30-min intervals for interstitial glucose variation during the three test days). ONE-way ANOVA was used to compare data at the single time points during the bread load, and T-Student's test for paired data was applied when appropriate. p values ≤ 0.05 were considered statistically significant. All statistics were performed with the SPSS software package V28 for Windows.

3. Results

3.1. Bread Characterisation

The three different kinds of bread were highly different in terms of glucose/fructose and lactic acid composition. Both the functional alkaline water bread and sourdough-leavened bread had a similar low concentration of glucose/fructose, which was somehow 10–15 times lower than the bakery yeast bread, while the sourdough-leavened bread was richer in lactic acid (Table 3).

Table 3. Moisture [weight loss in grams from 100 g of dough left for 5 h in an oven at 100 °C], simple carbohydrate, and lactic acid concentrations at the end of fermentation/maturation in the three different breads.

	Moisture [g]	Glucose g/100 g	Fructose g/100 g	Lactic Acid g/100 g
Functional alkaline water bread	32	0.062	0.1	<0.001
Sourdough-leavened bread	30	0.05	0.22	0.381
Bakery yeast bread	27	1.5	1.3	<0.001

Microbiological analysis showed the absence of bacterial growth on the plates belonging to the X and W doughs, while 100% of the colonies isolated from the plates of the sourdough (Y) dough belonged to *Pediococcus parvulus*. The absence of contamination was confirmed by the absence of bacterial growth on LB agar plates plated with suspensions of each dough.

3.2. Effect of the Different Bread Doughs on Interstitial Glucose, Capillary Blood Glucose, and Serum Insulin

Absolute changes (delta values) in interstitial glucose at 30-min intervals for all the observational periods were significantly higher with the bakery yeast bread (W) than the sourdough-leavened bread (Y) and functional alkaline water bread (X) after 60 min ($p < 0.05$ and $p < 0.01$, respectively), 90 min ($p < 0.05$ and $p < 0.01$, respectively), and 180 min ($p < 0.01$ for both). The peak glucose concentration was anticipated at 90′ with W compared to Y and X (120′ for both) (Figure 2).

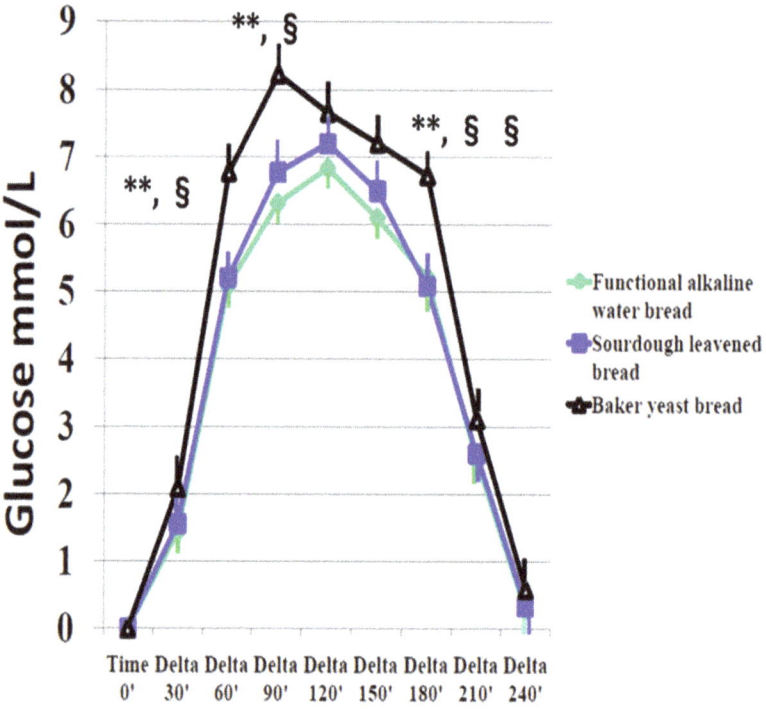

Figure 2. Interstitial glucose as determined by FGM in the 12 patients during the three different experimental days. Delta changes from basal in interstitial glucose determined at 30-min intervals during the entire experiment as determined by FGM. ** $p < 0.01$ functional alkaline water bread vs. bakery yeast bread; § $p < 0.05$. §§ $p < 0.01$ sourdough-leavened bread versus bakery yeast bread in the 12 T2DM.

The AUC of interstitial glucose as determined by Libre FGM in the period of 0–240 min was significantly higher with bakery yeast bread (W) in comparison to the other two tested breads, without a significant difference between these last two (Table 4). The interstitial glucose at time 0 and the peak glucose concentration were not significantly different from what was obtained when measuring blood glucose in the three different test days (Table 4). The delta peak blood glucose was significantly lower in the functional alkaline water bread and sourdough-leavened bread as compared to the bakery yeast bread ($p < 0.05$). No significant differences were evident for basal insulin in the three test days, while the insulin at peak glucose was significantly higher in the bakery yeast bread as compared to the functional alkaline water bread ($p < 0.05$) and sourdough-leavened bread ($p < 0.05$), without significant differences between the last two (Table 4).

Table 4. Effect of the different bread doughs in the twelve T2DM.

	X	Y	W	p
Interstitial Glucose mmol/L				
AUC 0–240 min	819.6 ± 72.1	926.0 ± 73.4	1016.4 ± 84.4	**,§
Time −10′	7.4 ± 0.5	7.3 ± 0.3	7.4 ± 0.5	ns
Delta peak/basal	7.7 ± 0.3	8.0 ± 0.9	9.4 ± 0.5	ns
Capillary blood glucose mmol/L				
Time −10′	7.3 ± 0.4	7.2 ± 0.3	7.3 ± 0.3	ns
Delta peak/basal	7.7 ± 0.4	8.1 ± 0.7	9.3 ± 0.6	*,^
Serum insulin [µU/mL]				
Basal insulin	9.5 ± 2.1	9.3 ± 1.9	9.7 ± 1.7	ns
Peak insulin	63.5 ± 10.8	62.2 ± 10.5	85.7 ± 14.2	*,§

AUC = area under the curve. Interstitial glucose: glucose determined by FGM; capillary blood glucose: glucose determined by finger prick test. X: functional alkaline water bread; Y: sourdough-leavened bread; W: bakery yeast bread. Data are means ± SEM. * $p < 0.05$, and ** $p < 0.01$ X vs. W; ^ $p < 0.05$, X vs. Y; § $p < 0.05$, Y vs. W. No significant differences were present within any group for both basal and peak glucose concentration measured in blood and determined by FGM.

No significant changes in the baseline anthropometric and biochemical data were present at the end of the three experimental days in the twelve T2DM. AGP reports were downloaded at the end of the 14 days, with either the mean glucose concentration (7.0 ± 0.1 mmol/L), the glucose management index (42 ± 1.3 mmol/L), or the time in range—TIR (80 ± 3.4%) confirming the good metabolic control of the twelve T2DM during the 14-day study period.

Additional material has been added at the end of the emanuscript (see Appendix A).

4. Discussion

A decreased postprandial glucose concentration induced by a low-GL diet is associated with a reduced risk for cardiovascular disease [26,27], particularly in persons with diabetes [28,29] and, likely, could help in preventing some forms of cancer [30,31]. In addition, low-carbohydrate [32–34] or low-GL diets [35,36] result in great weight loss over periods of 3–6 months and have a favorable effect on triglyceride and HDL cholesterol [37].

In this work, we analyzed the GL induced by three different breads, and we observed a significant decrease in GL induced by functional alkaline water bread and sourdough-leavened bread compared with bakery yeast bread. Although one limitation of this "acute" study is that the results cannot be transferred in the long term, these results suggest that the continuous use of these kinds of breads might be useful in reducing weight in overweight/obese T2DM when assumed chronically, with beneficial effects on both glycemic metabolic control and the reduction in cardiovascular risk. These results may encourage the commencement of long-term studies in this direction.

Interestingly, we also observed a reduction in postprandial blood glucose, a well-established cardiovascular risk factor in T2DM, with both the functional alkaline water and sourdough-leavened bread. Foods with high GI can result in an increase in blood glucose and insulin concentration in blood, whereas those with low GI do not have these effects [38], ultimately reducing the cardiovascular risk and diabetes onset in predisposed subjects.

In recent years, there has been an increased focus by food manufacturers on the use of low-glycemic products, replacing the sugars and starch in conventional food with ingredients such as alcohols, oligo- and polysaccharides, or glycerin. The effectiveness of added dietary fibers in reducing the GL of bread is controversial [39]. In addition, even if the inclusion of fibers or wholemeal flour in the production of bread can influence the glycemic response, the protocols to implement this method, to be effective, must consider the use of different technologies which are sometimes complicated to implement in practice [40]. Another method described for the reduction in GL in bread is the addition of beta glycans, [41], which effectively reduce GL, but their taste is not very pleasant and they are therefore not usable in practice. Other authors have suggested replacing breads with rice, potatoes, or hummus [42], but this option is difficult to apply to Mediterranean culture, where bread is one of the main sources of carbohydrates.

It has been reported that sourdough-leaved bread has a lower GI than commercial bread, due to the consumption of glucose by the enzymes of the lactobacilli bacterial and fungal flora of the dough " mother", improving glucose metabolism in healthy subjects [43]. This effect has been attributed mainly to the reduction in sugars and the presence of lactic acid. Previously, postprandial glycemic and insulinemic responses to a meal containing sourdough bread, compared to a reference meal containing leavened bread with yeast for bread making, in subjects with impaired glucose tolerance was evaluated [44]. A limitation of that study was that a 500-calorie mixed meal (100 g of bread, 200 mL of semi-skimmed milk, 15 g of glucose-free marmalade, 10 g of butter) containing 58% carbohydrates, 12% protein, and 30% lipids was used. The mixed meal might have altered the absorption of carbohydrates, making the interpretation of the data difficult.

In this study, we offered bread alone with a total of 480 calories to T2DM, and both the functional alkaline water and sourdough-leavened bread resulted in a lower AUC over the period of 240 min, together with a significantly lower increase in glucose at the predetermined 60, 90, and 180 min. Both kinds of breads had somehow 10–15-fold less simple sugar due to the consumption operated by lactobacilli in sourdough-leavened bread in a relatively short period and by yeasts operating for 48 h in functional alkaline water bread. The process of maturation in the functional water bread lasted between 24 and 48 h due to the fact that the starting pH was 9.0 and so remained ideal [pH 5.0] until the end of the maturation period. Without using the functional water, the pH of the dough would have rapidly gone below pH 3.0, making the dough inedible. Due to the similar results obtained with the two breads, we have hypothesized that the main driver of the reduction in glycemic response to the meal was the consumption of simple sugars more than the presence of lactic acid, although we cannot exclude the idea that the more complete maturation time obtained with the functional water bread might have influenced sugar absorption. Sourdough-leavened bread only had a significant amount of lactic acid, as expected by the presence of *Pediococcus parvolus*, a species belonging to lactic acid bacteria commonly associated with the fermentation process of wines and cider and recently found in sourdough of household origin [45].

Bakers and pizza makers choose to use rapid leavening dough since the use of "mother" yeast has very narrow margins of use, caused by the very tight fermentation/maturation time (between 6 and 8 h). This time affects the work activity of the baker, with repercussions on the final price and therefore causing a reduction in the possibility of spreading this type of dough to the general population. A much more flexible process that could foresee a leavening/maturation time with wider margins, between 24 and 48 h at room temperature, would clearly allow the baker to lower costs and therefore the increase the possibility of greater diffusion at the population level. We found no bacterial growth in our "functional" bread, indicating that the process of maturation/leaving for 48 h at room temperature is safe.

To the best of our knowledge, this is the first time that FGM has been used to determine glucose variations in response to different doughs in humans. We measured blood glucose and insulin by finger pricks at both basal and peak interstitial glucose concentrations in a moment when the two compartments were in equilibrium, with no significant differences between blood and interstitial glucose. On the other hand, using the plot of the curve of interstitial glucose variation over 240 min after eating the bread, we were able to calculate the AUC by the trapezoidal rule at 5-min intervals, giving a more precise calculation compared to what is usually determined at 30-min intervals. Using FGM, we were also able to observe the glucose patterns in the days before the three experiments and, in particular, the night before.

One limitation of this study is that the results cannot be transferred in the long term, being an "acute"study. Long-term population studies could favor the production of this kind of bread at the same cost as regular bread, allowing to diffuse it amongst the whole population, prioritizing the health of the general population with a "small coin for big numbers". At present, we are trying to start this implementation in the local population.

5. Conclusions

(1) Bread prepared with biocrystal water has the same low glycemic load of sourdough bread compared to traditional bread, and it enables the easier management of the leavening/maturation period.
(2) FGM is a reliable method to determine the area under the curve during glycemic changes in response to a carbohydrate meal in persons with type 2 diabetes.

Author Contributions: M.A.T. and G.T. initiated and designed the study; M.A.T., G.T. and S.C. performed the experiments; V.M., G.C. and P.R. collected and performed the microbiological analysis; S.C. prepared the balanced diets for the twelve T2DM and performed insulin measurements; I.C. collected and analyzed the data; G.T. and M.A.T. analyzed and interpreted the data and wrote the initial draft of the manuscript. All authors critically reviewed the manuscript through the process and approved the final draft of the manuscript. All authors have read and agreed to the published version of the manuscript.

Funding: This research received no external funding.

Institutional Review Board Statement: "COMITATO BIOETICA ATS SARDEGNA" on 14 July 2020 (NP 248/2020/CE).

Informed Consent Statement: Informed consent was obtained from all subjects involved in the study.

Data Availability Statement: The raw data supporting the conclusions of this article will be made available by the authors on request.

Acknowledgments: We thank Fabrizio Contino, for sharing his idea regarding the functional biocrystal alkaline water and for preparing the different doughs. We thank JANASDIA (Associazione Scientifica Ricerca sul Diabete ONLUS, www.janasdia.com, accessed on 5 August 2021) for covering the expense of the insulin determinations, biochemical analyses, and FGM sensors for the patients.

Conflicts of Interest: The authors declare that they have no conflicts of interest.

Appendix A

Table A1. Randomization chart.

Patient	SEX	Test Day 1	Test Day 2	Test Day 3
1	M	X	Y	W
2	F	X	Y	W
3	M	X	Y	W
4	F	W	X	Y
5	M	W	X	Y
6	M	W	X	Y
7	F	Y	W	X
8	M	Y	W	X
9	M	Y	W	X
10	F	W	Y	X
11	F	Y	X	Y
12	F	X	W	W

M = male, F = female; X = functional alkaline water bread; Y = sourdough-leavened bread; W = bakery yeast bread. Tests were performed in single-blind conditions on three different days in random order, three days apart, over a period of two weeks.

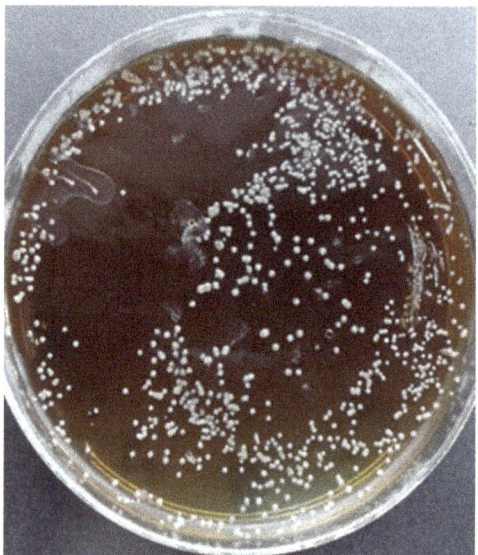

Figure A1. Colonies of lactic acid bacteria obtained from sourdough-leavened bread dough sample (Y).

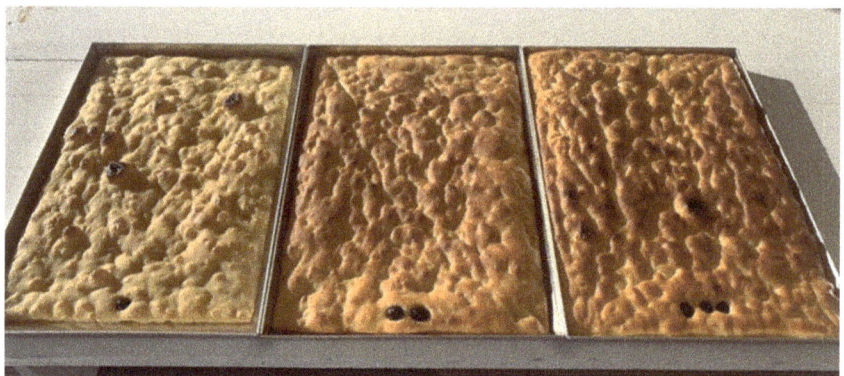

Figure A2. Appearance of the different types of bread after baking and immediately before serving. The three different types of bread as they were prepared for each session from left to right: functional alkaline water bread, sourdough-leavened bread, bakery yeast bread.

Table A2. Results from the 5-point hedonic scale for each sensorial attribute.

Bread	Smell	Taste	Consistency	Acceptance
Functional alkaline water bread	3.9 ± 1.1	4.1 ± 1.1	4.4 ± 0.9	4.6 ± 0.5
Sourdough-leavened bread	4.7 ± 0.4 *	4.7 ± 0.4	4.7 ± 0.7	4.8 ± 0.3
Bakery yeast bread	4.2 ± 1.2	4.3 ± 1.0	4.6 ± 0.7	4.7 ± 0.5

* $p < 0.05$ vs. functional alkaline water bread. To determine consumer acceptability, a simple 5-point hedonic scale questionnaire for each sensorial attribute (odor, taste, texture, and general acceptance during the test) was used, where 5 was the highest score (i.e., extremely positive = like very much) and 1 the lowest (i.e., extremely negative = dislike very much). No substantial differences in terms of the consumer acceptability of the three different bread were reported apart from smell.

References

1. Jenkins, D.J.; Wolever, T.M.; Taylor, R.H.; Barker, H.; Fielden, H.; Baldwin, J.M.; Bowling, A.C.; Newman, H.C.; Jenkins, A.L.; Goff, D.V. Glycemic index of foods: A physiological basis for carbohydrate exchange. *Am. J. Clin. Nutr.* **1981**, *34*, 362–366. [CrossRef] [PubMed]
2. Wolever, T.M.S.; Jenkins, D. The use of the glycemic index in predicting the blood glucose response to mixed meals. *Am. J. Clin. Nutr.* **1986**, *43*, 167–172. [CrossRef] [PubMed]
3. Coutinho, M.; Gerstein, H.C.; Wang, Y.; Yusuf, S. Relationship between glucose and incident cardiovascular events. A metaregression analysis of published data from 20 studies of 95,783 individuals followed for 12.4 years. *Diabetes Care* **1999**, *22*, 233–240. [CrossRef] [PubMed]
4. Levitan, E.B.; Song, Y.; Ford, E.S.; Liu, S. Is non diabetic hyperglycemia a risk factor for cardiovascular disease? A meta-analysis of prospective studies. *Arch. Intern. Med.* **2004**, *164*, 2147–2155. [CrossRef] [PubMed]
5. Glucose tolerance and mortality: Comparison of WHO and American Diabetes Association diagnostic criteria. The DECODE study group.European Diabetes Epidemiology Group, Glucose tolerance and mortality: Comparison of WHO and American Diabetes Association diagnostic criteria. Diabetes Epidemiology: Collaborative analysis of Diagnostic criteria in Europe. *Lancet* **1999**, *354*, 617–621. [CrossRef]
6. Vega-López, S.; Mayol-Kreiser, S.N. Use of the glycemic index for weight loss and glycemic control: A review of recent evidence. *Curr. Diabetes Rep.* **2009**, *9*, 379–388. [CrossRef]
7. Zelenskiy, S.; Thompson, C.L.; Tucker, T.C.; Li, L. High dietary glycemic load is associated with increased risk of colon cancer. *Nutr. Cancer* **2014**, *66*, 362–368. [CrossRef]
8. Parker, A.; Kim, Y. The Effect of Low Glycemic Index and Glycemic Load Diets on Hepatic Fat Mass, Insulin Resistance, and Blood Lipid Panels in Individuals with Nonalcoholic Fatty Liver Disease. *Metab. Syndr. Relat. Disord.* **2019**, *17*, 389–396. [CrossRef]
9. Schwingshackl, L.; Hoffmann, G. Long-term effects of low glycemic index/load vs. high glycemic index/load diets on parameters of obesity and obesity-associated risks: A systematic review and meta-analysis. *Nutr. Metab. Cardiovasc. Dis.* **2013**, *23*, 699–706. [CrossRef]
10. Capurso, A.; Capurso, C. The Mediterranean way: Why elderly people should eat wholewheat sourdough bread—A little known component of the Mediterranean diet and healthy food for elderly adults. *Aging Clin. Exp. Res.* **2020**, *32*, 1–5. [CrossRef]
11. Sterr, Y.; Weiss, A.; Schmidt, H. Evaluation of lactic acid bacteria for sourdough fermentation of amaranth. *Int. J. Food Microbiol.* **2009**, *136*, 75–82. [CrossRef] [PubMed]
12. Montemurro, M.; Coda, R.; Rizzello, C.G. Recent Advances in the Use of Sourdough Biotechnology in Pasta Making. *Foods* **2019**, *8*, 129. [CrossRef] [PubMed]
13. Daugirdas, J.T. Potential importance of low-sodium bread and breakfast cereal to a reduced sodium diet. *J. Ren. Nutr.* **2013**, *23*, 1–3. [CrossRef] [PubMed]
14. Cappon, G.; Vettoretti, M.; Sparacino, G.; Facchinetti, A. Continuous Glucose Monitoring Sensors for Diabetes Management: A Review of Technologies and Applications. *Diabetes Metab. J.* **2019**, *43*, 383–397. [CrossRef] [PubMed]
15. Bailey, T.; Bode, B.W.; Christiansen, M.P.; Klaff, L.J.; Alva, S. The performance and usability of a factory-calibrated flash glucose monitoring system. *Diabetes Technol. Ther.* **2015**, *17*, 787–794. [CrossRef] [PubMed]
16. Giani, E.; Macedoni, M.; Barilli, A.; Petitti, A.; Mameli, C.; Bosetti, A.; Cristiano, A.; Radovanovic, D.; Santus, P.; Zuccotti, G.V. Performance of the flash glucose monitoring system during exercise in youth with type 1 diabetes. *Diabetes Res. Clin. Pract.* **2018**, *146*, 321–329. [CrossRef] [PubMed]
17. Blum, A. Freestyle Libre glucose monitoring system. *Clin. Diabetes* **2018**, *36*, 203–204. [CrossRef]
18. Hayek, A.A.; Al Dawish, M.A. The Potential Impact of the FreeStyle Libre Flash Glucose Monitoring System on Mental Well-Being and Treatment satisfaction in patients with type 1 diabetes: A prospective study. *Diabetes Ther.* **2019**, *10*, 1239–1248. [CrossRef]
19. Ji, L.; Guo, X.; Guo, L.; Ren, Q.; Yu, N.; Zhang, J. A multicenter evaluation of the performance and usability of a novel glucose monitoring system in Chinese adults with diabetes. *J. Diabetes Sci. Technol.* **2017**, *11*, 290–295. [CrossRef]
20. Ang, E.; Lee, Z.X.; Moore, S.; Nana, M. Flash glucose monitoring [FGM]: A clinical review on glycaemic outcomes and impact on quality of life. *J. Diabetes Its Complicat.* **2020**, *34*, 107559. [CrossRef]
21. Lévesque, S.; Dufresne, P.J.; Soualhine, H.; Domingo, M.-C.; Bekal, S.; Lefebvre, B.; Tremblay, C. A side by side comparison of Bruker Biotyper and VITEK MS: Utility of MALDI-TOF MS technology for microorganism identification in a public health reference laboratory. *PLoS ONE* **2015**, *10*, e0144878. [CrossRef] [PubMed]
22. Westblade, L.F.; Jennemann, R.; Branda, J.A.; Bythrow, M.; Ferraro, M.J.; Garner, O.B.; Ginocchio, C.C.; Lewinski, M.A.; Manji, R.; Mochon, A.B.; et al. Multicenter study evaluating the Vitek MS system for identification of medically important yeasts. *J. Clin. Microbiol.* **2013**, *51*, 2267–2272. [CrossRef] [PubMed]
23. Ghaith, D.; Zafer, M.M.; Hosny, T.; AbdElfattah, M. MALDI-TOF MS Overcomes Misidentification of the Uncommon Human Pathogen Candida famata by Routine Phenotypic Identification Methods. *Curr. Microbiol.* **2021**, *78*, 1636–1642. [CrossRef] [PubMed]
24. Yari, Z.; Behrouz, V.; Zand, H.; Pourvali, K. New Insight into Diabetes Management: From Glycemic Index to Dietary Insulin Index. *Curr. Diabetes Rev.* **2020**, *16*, 293–300. [CrossRef]

25. Matthews, D.R.; Hosker, J.P.; Rudenski, A.S.; Naylor, B.A.; Treacher, D.F.; Turner, R.C. Homeostasis model assessment: Insulin resistance and beta-cell function from fasting plasma glucose and insulin concentrations in man. *Diabetologia* **1985**, *28*, 412–419. [CrossRef] [PubMed]
26. Liu, S.; Willett, W.C.; Stampfer, M.J.; Hu, F.B.; Franz, M.; Sampson, L.; Hennekens, C.H.; Manson, J.E. A prospective study of dietary glycemic load, carbohydrate intake and risk of coronary heart disease in US women. *Am. J. Clin. Nutr.* **2000**, *71*, 1455–1461. [CrossRef] [PubMed]
27. Frost, G.; Leeds, A.A.; Dore, C.J.; Madeiros, S.; Brading, S.; Dornhorst, A. Glycaemic index as a determinant of serum HDL-cholesterol concentration. *Lancet* **1999**, *353*, 1045–1048. [CrossRef]
28. Salmerón, J.; Ascherio, A.; Rimm, E.B.; A Colditz, G.; Spiegelman, D.; Jenkins, D.J.; Stampfer, M.J.; Wing, A.L.; Willett, W.C. Dietary fiber, glycemic load, and risk of NIDDM in men. *Diabetes Care* **1997**, *20*, 545–550. [CrossRef]
29. Salmerón, J.; Manson, J.E.; Stampfer, M.J.; Colditz, G.A.; Wing, A.L.; Willett, W.C. Dietary fiber, glycemic load and risk of non-insulin dependent diabetes mellitus in women. *JAMA* **1997**, *277*, 472–477. [CrossRef]
30. Augustin, L.S.A.; Dal Maso, L.; La Vecchia, C.; Parpinel, M.; Negri, E.; Vaccarella, S.; Kendall, C.W.C.; Jenkins, D.J.A.; Franceschi, S. Dietary glycemic index and glycemic load, and breast cancer risk: A case-control study. *Ann. Oncol.* **2001**, *12*, 1533–1538. [CrossRef]
31. Higginbotham, S.; Zhang, Z.-F.; Lee, I.-M.; Cook, N.R.; Giovannucci, E.; Buring, J.E.; Liu, S. Women's Health Study Dietary glycemic load and risk of colorectal cancer in the Women's Health Study. *J. Natl. Cancer Inst.* **2004**, *96*, 229–233. [CrossRef] [PubMed]
32. Foster, G.D.; Wyatt, H.R.; Hill, J.O.; McGuckin, B.G.; Brill, C.; Mohammed, B.S.; Szapary, P.O.; Rader, D.J.; Edman, J.S.; Klein, S. A randomized trial of a low-carbohydrate diet for obesity. *N. Engl. J. Med.* **2003**, *348*, 2082–2090. [CrossRef] [PubMed]
33. Westman, E.C.; Yancy, W.S.; Edman, J.S.; Tomlin, K.F.; E Perkins, C. Effect of 6-Month Adherence to a Very Low Carbohydrate Diet Program. *Am. J. Med.* **2002**, *113*, 30–36. [CrossRef] [PubMed]
34. Samaha, F.F.; Iqbal, N.; Seshadri, P.; Chicano, K.L.; Daily, D.A.; McGrory, J.; Williams, T.; Williams, M.; Gracely, E.J.; Stern, L. A low-carbohydrate as compared with a low-fat diet in severe obesity. *N. Engl. J. Med.* **2003**, *348*, 2074–2081. [CrossRef]
35. Ebbeling, C.B.; Leidig, M.M.; Sinclair, K.B.; Hangen, J.P.; Ludwig, D.S. A reduced-glycemic load diet in the treatment of adolescent obesity. *Arch. Pediatr. Adolesc. Med.* **2003**, *157*, 773–779. [CrossRef] [PubMed]
36. McMillan-Price, J.; Petocz, P.; Atkinson, F.; O'neill, K.; Samman, S.; Steinbeck, K.; Caterson, I.; Brand-Miller, J. Comparison of 4 diets of varying glycemic load on weight loss and cardiovascular risk reduction in overweight and obese young adults: A randomized controlled trial. *Arch. Intern. Med.* **2006**, *166*, 1466–1475. [CrossRef] [PubMed]
37. Stern, L.; Iqbal, N.; Seshadri, P.; Chicano, K.L.; Daily, D.A.; McGrory, J.; Williams, M.; Gracely, E.J.; Samaha, F.F. The Effects of Low-Carbohydrate versus Conventional Weight Loss Diets in Severely Obese Adults: One-Year Follow-up of a Randomized Trial. *Ann. Intern. Med.* **2004**, *140*, 778–785. [CrossRef]
38. Wolever, T.M.; Jenkins, D.J.; Jenkins, A.L.; Josse, R.G. The glycemic index: Methodology and clinical implications. *Am. J. Clin. Nutr.* **1991**, *54*, 846–854. [CrossRef]
39. Scazzina, F.; Siebenhandl-Ehn, S.; Pellegrini, N. The effect of dietary fibre on reducing the glycaemic index of bread. *Br. J. Nutr.* **2013**, *109*, 1163–1174. [CrossRef]
40. Korem, T.; Zeevi, D.; Zmora, N.; Weissbrod, O.; Bar, N.; Lotan-Pompan, M.; Avnit-Sagi, T.; Kosower, N.; Malka, G.; Rein, M.; et al. Bread Affects Clinical Parameters and Induces Gut Microbiome-Associated Personal Glycemic Responses. *Cell Metab.* **2017**, *25*, 1243–1253.e5. [CrossRef]
41. Tessari, P.; Lante, A. A Multifunctional Bread Rich in Beta Glucans and Low in Starch Improves Metabolic Control in Type 2 Diabetes: A Controlled Trial. *Nutrients* **2017**, *9*, 297. [CrossRef]
42. Augustin, L.S.A.; Chiavaroli, L.; Campbell, J.; Ezatagha, A.; Jenkins, A.L.; Esfahani, A.; Kendall, C.W.C. Post-prandial glucose and insulin responses of hummus alone or combined with a carbohydrate food: A dose—Response study. *Nutr. J.* **2016**, *15*, 13. [CrossRef]
43. Ostman, E.M.; Elmståhl, H.G.M.L.; Björck, I.M.E. Barley Bread containing lactid acid improves glucose tolerance at a subsequent meal in healthy men and women. *J. Nutr.* **2002**, *132*, 1173–1175. [CrossRef]
44. Maioli, M.; Pes, G.M.; Sanna, M.; Cherchi, S.; Dettori, M.; Manca, E.; Farris, G.A. Sourdough-leavened Bread Improves Postprandial Glucose and Insulin Plasma Levels in Subjects with Impaired Glucose Tolerance. *Acta Diabetol.* **2008**, *45*, 91–96. [CrossRef]
45. Comasio, A.; Verce, M.; Van Kerrebroeck, S.; De Vuyst, L. Diverse Microbial Composition of Sourdoughs from Different Origins. *Front. Microbiol.* **2020**, *11*, 1212. [CrossRef] [PubMed]

Disclaimer/Publisher's Note: The statements, opinions and data contained in all publications are solely those of the individual author(s) and contributor(s) and not of MDPI and/or the editor(s). MDPI and/or the editor(s) disclaim responsibility for any injury to people or property resulting from any ideas, methods, instructions or products referred to in the content.

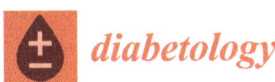

Communication

Effectiveness of Oral versus Injectable Semaglutide in Adults with Type 2 Diabetes: Results from a Retrospective Observational Study in Croatia

Sanja Klobučar [1,2,*], Andrej Belančić [3,4], Iva Bukša [5], Nikolina Morić [6] and Dario Rahelić [7,8,9]

1. Department of Internal Medicine, Division of Endocrinology, Diabetes and Metabolic Diseases, Clinical Hospital Centre Rijeka, 51000 Rijeka, Croatia
2. Department of Internal Medicine, Faculty of Medicine, University of Rijeka, 51000 Rijeka, Croatia
3. Department of Clinical Pharmacology, Clinical Hospital Centre Rijeka, 51000 Rijeka, Croatia; a.belancic93@gmail.com or andrej.belancic@uniri.hr
4. Department of Basic and Clinical Pharmacology with Toxicology, Faculty of Medicine, University of Rijeka, 51000 Rijeka, Croatia
5. Department of Urology, Clinical Hospital Centre Rijeka, 51000 Rijeka, Croatia; ivabuksa@gmail.com
6. Health Center of Primorje–Gorski Kotar County, 51000 Rijeka, Croatia; nikolinamorich@gmail.com
7. Vuk Vrhovac University Clinic for Diabetes, Endocrinology and Metabolic Diseases, Merkur University Hospital, 10000 Zagreb, Croatia; dario.rahelic@gmail.com
8. School of Medicine, Catholic University of Croatia, 10000 Zagreb, Croatia
9. Faculty of Medicine, J.J. Strossmayer University Osijek, 31000 Osijek, Croatia
* Correspondence: sanja.klobucar@uniri.hr

Abstract: Background: The number of people with type 2 diabetes is increasing daily, and therefore, effective therapy is needed to successfully regulate glycemia and reduce the risk of associated complications. Recently, an oral formulation of the glucagon-like peptide-1 receptor agonist (GLP-1 RA) semaglutide has become available. Therefore, the aim of our study was to compare the effectiveness of the new oral formulation and the existing injectable formulation of semaglutide in terms of glycemic and body weight control in a real-world setting. Patients and methods: This was a single-center retrospective observational study conducted at the Rijeka Clinical Hospital Centre. A total of 106 patients with inadequately controlled type 2 diabetes (HbA1c ≥ 7%) on different oral or basal insulin supported oral therapy were enrolled in the study, and data from electronic medical records were retrospectively collected and analyzed from May 2021 to November 2022. All subjects were GLP-1 RA-naive and consequently prescribed 0.5 or 1.0 mg of once weekly injectable semaglutide (IS) or 7 mg or 14 mg of once daily oral semaglutide (OS) for at least 6 months. Glycated hemoglobin (HbA1c), body weight, and body mass index (BMI) were assessed prior to semaglutide administration and after a 6-month follow-up period. The primary endpoint was the change from baseline in HbA1c, and secondary endpoints were the change in body weight and the proportion of participants with a reduction in body weight of ≥5% and ≥10%, respectively, 6 months after the initiation of semaglutide treatment. Results: At the 6-month follow-up, no significant difference was observed between the two formulations in terms of HbA1c reduction (IS −1.1% vs. OS −1.4%, $p = 0.126$) and weight loss (IS −6.50 kg vs. OS −5.90 kg, $p = 0.714$). Exactly the same proportion of participants in both groups achieved a weight loss of ≥5% (56.7%, n = 30). A weight loss ≥ 10% was observed in 20.7% (n = 11) of participants administered IS and 15.1% (n = 8) of participants administered OS, respectively ($p = 0.454$). Conclusion: In a real-world setting, oral semaglutide as an add-on therapy to ongoing antihyperglycemic treatment in patients with inadequately controlled type 2 diabetes who had not previously received GLP-1 RA demonstrated a similar effectiveness as injectable semaglutide in terms of glycemic control and weight loss after 6 months of treatment.

Keywords: glucagon-like peptide-1; semaglutide; type 2 diabetes

Citation: Klobučar, S.; Belančić, A.; Bukša, I.; Morić, N.; Rahelić, D. Effectiveness of Oral versus Injectable Semaglutide in Adults with Type 2 Diabetes: Results from a Retrospective Observational Study in Croatia. *Diabetology* 2024, 5, 60–68. https://doi.org/10.3390/diabetology5010005

Academic Editor: Peter Clifton

Received: 28 August 2023
Revised: 18 December 2023
Accepted: 19 January 2024
Published: 2 February 2024

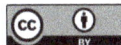

Copyright: © 2024 by the authors. Licensee MDPI, Basel, Switzerland. This article is an open access article distributed under the terms and conditions of the Creative Commons Attribution (CC BY) license (https://creativecommons.org/licenses/by/4.0/).

1. Introduction

According to International Diabetes Federation, it is estimated that 537 million people worldwide have diabetes, and the vast majority of cases are type 2 diabetes (T2D). In addition, there are around 541 million people who have impaired glucose tolerance. It is predicted that by 2045, the number of diabetes cases will reach 783 million. By all accounts, diabetes is certainly one of the fastest-growing global health issues of the 21st century [1].

According to a recent systematic review, the leading cause of mortality and comorbidity in people with diabetes is cardiovascular disease (CVD), which accounts for 50.3% of all deaths [2]. It is assessed that in the U.S., around USD 37.3 billion per year is spent on treating cardiovascular-related complications associated with diabetes [3]. A great number of people with type 2 diabetes have cardiometabolic risk factors that can be modified, such as diet, smoking, sedentary lifestyle, dyslipidemia, hypertension, and obesity.

Clinical guidelines recommend an approach to the management of type 2 diabetes that goes beyond simply lowering glucose levels to reduce modifiable cardiometabolic risk factors [4–8]. Treatment should be guided by a person-centered, holistic, multifactorial approach that takes into account individual goals related to glycemic control, body weight, and cardiovascular risk factor management to maintain and improve patient well-being. It is well established that obesity significantly increases the risk of developing type 2 diabetes and is associated with numerous other psychosocial and medical complications [9,10].

According to the American Diabetes Association (ADA), overweight patients with T2D may benefit from modest weight loss (3–7% of baseline weight) in terms of improved glycemic management and cardiovascular risk factor improvement. Greater benefit, including improvement in long-term cardiovascular outcomes and possible remission of disease, results from sustained weight loss of greater than 10% of body weight. It is recommended that the potential beneficial effects on body weight be considered when choosing an antihyperglycemic drug. Pharmacological therapy for obesity in these patients is considered effective if the patient loses $\geq$ 5% of body weight after 3 months of therapy [9].

Over the past decade, a number of clinical trials have been published with results showing that modern therapies, including glucagon-like peptide-1 receptor agonists (GLP-1 RA) and SGLT-2 inhibitors, achieve significant and consistent cardiometabolic benefits [11]. GLP-1 RAs have been shown to be an effective treatment for patients with type 2 diabetes. Remarkable clinical benefits of GLP-1 RAs have been demonstrated, not only in maintaining glycemic control and protecting against hypoglycemia, but also in significant weight loss, lowering blood pressure, and improving lipid profiles [12]. Moreover, their use has been associated with a reduced risk of major cardiovascular events (MACE), cardiovascular death, nonfatal myocardial infarction, and nonfatal ischemic stroke in patients with T2D [13].

Semaglutide is the only GLP-1 RA available in both injectable and oral formulation. Impaired absorption of orally administered peptides has been overcome by co-formulation with the absorption enhancer sodium N-(8-[2 hydroxybenzoyl]amino)caprylate (SNAC) which protects semaglutide through local buffering and leads to facilitated absorption across the gastric epithelium [14,15]. The first oral formulation of GLP-1 RA semaglutide (Rybelsus) was approved by the U.S. Food and Drug Administration (FDA) in September 2019 and by European Medicines Agency (EMA) in April 2020 [16,17]. Due to the lower bioavailability of oral semaglutide compared to the subcutaneous formulation, a higher dose of 7 mg to 14 mg/day versus 1 mg to 2 mg/week of the subcutaneous formulation is required [18].

The efficacy of once-weekly subcutaneously administered semaglutide and once-daily oral semaglutide has been evaluated in the comprehensive clinical trial programs SUSTAIN and PIONEER. Both formulations of semaglutide have been shown to be nearly equally effective in achieving and maintaining glycemic targets, with 66–80% of participants administered semaglutide 1.0 mg subcutaneously achieving an HbA1c < 7% in SUSTAIN trials, compared with 55–77% of participants treated with oral semaglutide 14 mg throughout the PIONEER study program [19]. Moreover, the safety profile of both formulations is highly similar, and they have also been associated with significant weight loss and low risk of hypoglycemia [19].

However, to date, no direct comparative studies between injectable and oral semaglutide formulations have been performed evaluating their effects on glycemic control and body weight. Therefore, the aim of our study was to compare the effectiveness of the two semaglutide formulations in terms of glycemic and body weight control in a real-world setting.

2. Materials and Methods

2.1. Study Design and Population

This was a single-center retrospective observational study conducted at the Rijeka Clinical Hospital Centre. A total of 106 adult (>18 years of age) patients with inadequately controlled type 2 diabetes (HbA1c $\geq$ 7%) on different oral or basal insulin supported oral therapy were enrolled in the study. All subjects were GLP-1 RA-naive and consequently prescribed 0.5 or 1.0 mg of once weekly injectable semaglutide (IS) or 7 mg or 14 mg of once daily oral semaglutide (OS) for at least 6 months. Glycated hemoglobin (HbA1c), body weight, and body mass index (BMI) were assessed prior to semaglutide administration and after a 6-month follow-up period. The primary endpoint was the change from baseline in HbA1c, and secondary endpoints were the change in body weight and the proportion of participants with a reduction in body weight of $\geq$5% and $\geq$10%, respectively, 6 months after the initiation of semaglutide treatment. The study was conducted according to the guidelines of the Declaration of Helsinki and approved by the Institutional Review Board of Clinical Hospital Center Rijeka (No: 003-05/20-1/54).

2.2. Data Collection

Data from electronic medical records were retrospectively collected and analyzed from May 2021 to November 2022. Demographic (age, gender) and relevant clinical data [body weight, body height, BMI, HbA1c, comorbidities (arterial hypertension, dyslipidemia, cardio/cerebrovascular disease)] were collected.

2.3. Statistical Analysis

Statistical analysis was performed using Microsoft Excel 2016 for Windows, version is 1.0 (Microsoft Office) and MedCalc v12.1.3 (MedCalc Software bvba, Ostend, Belgium). Absolute and relative frequencies, measures of central tendency, and measures of spread were used to present the data. The Mann–Whitney test and the χ^2-test were used to compare outcomes between groups. Criterion for statistical significance was estimated on $p < 0.05$. All tests were run under 95% confidence interval (CI).

3. Results

The group of patients administered injectable semaglutide consisted of a total of 53 participants, 30 of whom were men and 23 women, aged 38–78 years. In this group, 10 (18.9%) patients received 0.5 mg of injectable semaglutide, and 43 (81.1%) of them received 1.0 mg. In addition, 12 (22.6%) patients were found to have cardiovascular disease (CVD). In addition to injectable semaglutide, patients also received previously prescribed concomitant therapy, including 48 (90.6%) metformin, 21 (39.6%) SGLT-2i, 11 (20.8%) a sulfonylurea, 3 (5.7%) pioglitazone, and 16 (30.2%) insulin.

The other group of patients who received oral semaglutide consisted of a total of 53 patients, 30 men and 23 women, aged 46–79 years. In this group, 20 (37.7%) patients received an oral semaglutide dose of 7 mg and 14 (62.3%) of them received a dose of 14 mg. CVD was confirmed in nine (17%) participants in this group. In addition to oral semaglutide, patients in this group also received previously prescribed concomitant therapy, 52 (98.1%) of them metformin, 24 (45.2%) patients SGLT-2i, 13 (24.5%) patients in therapy had a sulfonylurea, 2 (3.8%) patients pioglitazone, and 12 (22.6%) of them insulin.

The demographic and clinical characteristics of the patients (n = 106; 56.6% female), who were divided into two groups based on the therapy administered, are shown in Table 1. There were no significant differences between the oral semaglutide group and the injectable semaglutide group in age and confirmed cardiovascular disease (CVD). There was a difference between the doses of the investigational drugs (lower vs. upper dose) between the groups, in favor of the IS group ($p = 0.014$).

Table 1. Demographic and clinical characteristics of patients.

Variables	Injectable Semaglutide	Oral Semaglutide	p-Value
Number of patients (n)	53	53	
Male	56.6% (n = 30)	56.6% (n = 30)	
Female	43.4% (n = 23)	43.4% (n = 23)	
Age (years) *	63 (38–78)	59 (46–79)	0.552
Dosage (mg)	0.5 mg 18.9% (n = 10)	7 mg 37.7% (n = 20)	0.014 [a]
	1.0 mg 81.1% (n = 43)	14 mg 62.3% (n = 33)	
Confirmed CVD	22.6% (n = 12)	17% (n = 9)	0.095
Background therapy			
metformin	90.6% (n = 48)	98.1% (n = 52)	
SGLT-2i	39.6% (n = 21)	45.2% (n = 24)	
sulfonylurea	20.8% (n = 11)	24.5% (n = 13)	
pioglitazone	5.7% (n = 3)	3.8% (n = 2)	
insulin	30.2% (n = 16)	22.6% (n = 12)	

* Data are reported as median and interquartile range. [a] Categorical variables are analyzed with the Chi-Square (χ^2) test; $p < 0.05$.

Baseline HbA1c levels are shown in Figure 1. There was a difference in baseline HbA1c values between the injectable semaglutide group and the oral semaglutide group [median 8.0 (5.5–12.7 range) versus 8.80 (6.2–14.2)%, $p = 0.039$].

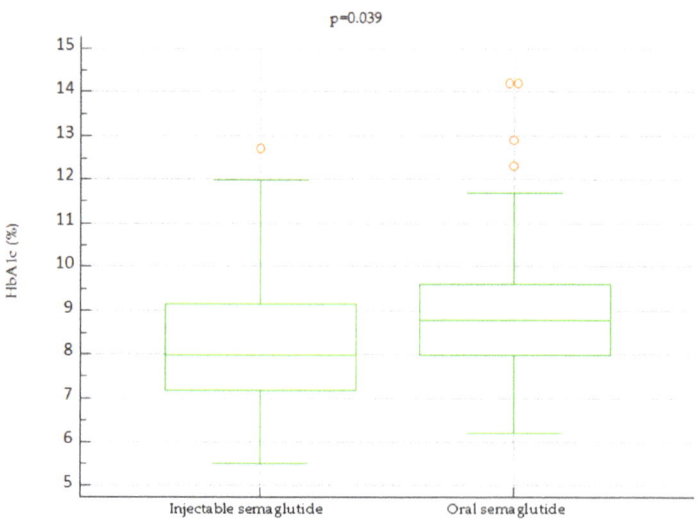

Figure 1. Box plot with comparisons of baseline HbA1c between IS and OS group.

There was no difference in terms of baseline body weight between the groups [mean 102.0 ± 5.1 kg standard deviation vs. 97.3 ± 5.9 kg ($p = 0.081$)] (Figure 2).

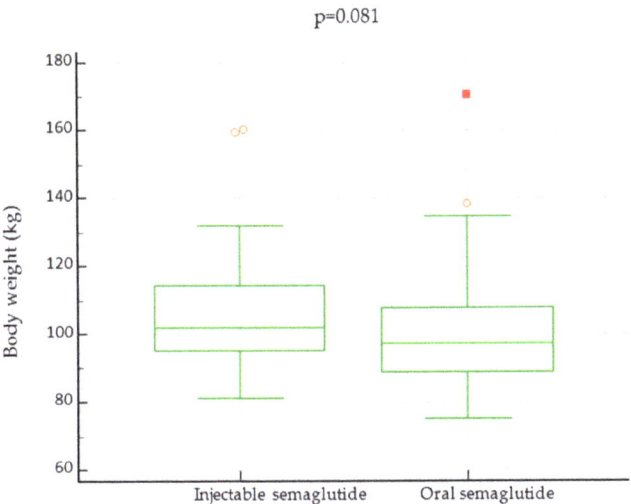

Figure 2. Box plot with comparisons of baseline body weight between IS and OS group.

In addition, no difference was found between groups in baseline BMI [median 34.72 (27.41–46.61 range) vs. 32.87 (25.73–51.45) kg/m^2, $p = 0.185$] (Figure 3).

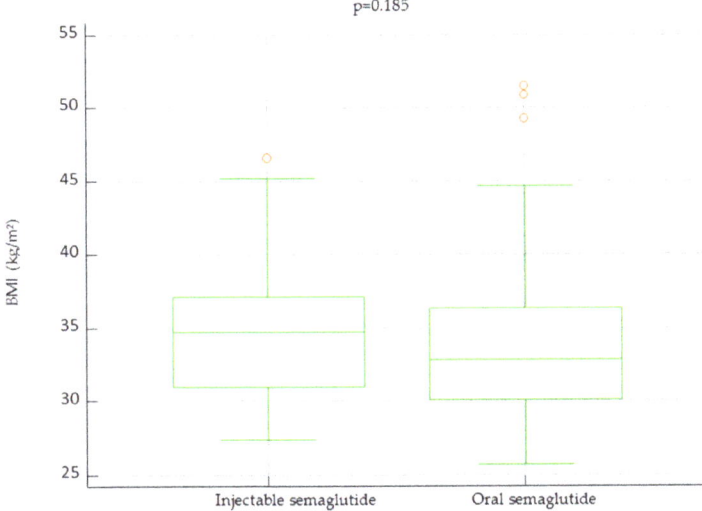

Figure 3. Box plot with comparisons of baseline body mass index between IS and OS group.

When comparing the efficacy of IS and OS in lowering blood glucose (using HbA1c as a surrogate), no difference was observed between the two formulations at 6 months [-median 1.10 (−7.10–4.60 range) vs. −1.40 (−8.0–0.70)%, $p = 0.126$] (Figure 4).

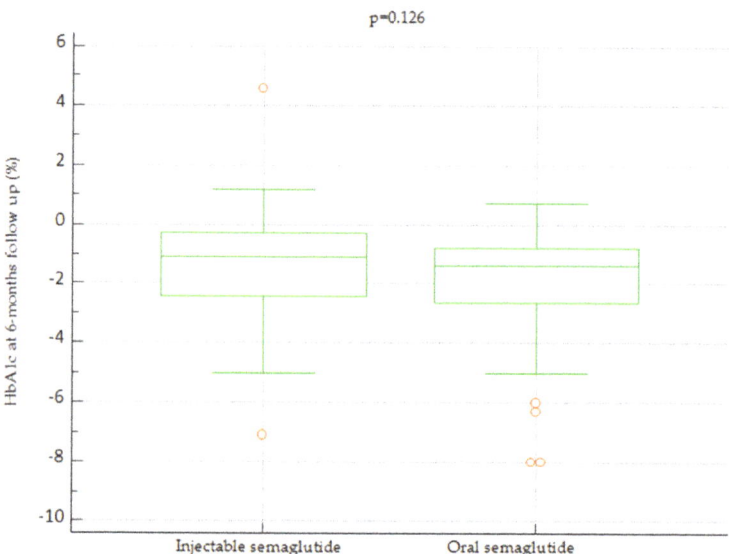

Figure 4. Change in HbA1c after 6 month of treatment with IS vs. OS.

At 6-month follow-up, no difference in body weight was observed between the injectable semaglutide group and the oral semaglutide group [median −6.50 (−28.0–10.0 range) vs. −5.90 (−45.3–0.2) kg, $p = 0.714$], as shown in Figure 5.

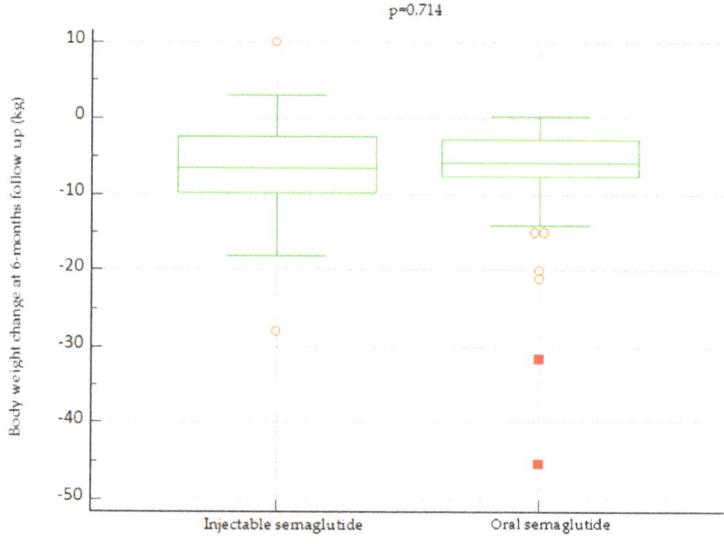

Figure 5. Change in body weight after 6 month of treatment with IS vs. OS.

Participants in both groups, 56.7% in total (n = 30), achieved a loss of body mass of >5% with no difference between groups. Weight loss of > 10% was observed in 20.7% (n = 11) of patients on injectable semaglutide and in 15.1% (n = 8) of patients on oral semaglutide, with no difference between the groups.

The most common adverse side effect was nausea, which was generally mild to moderate and transient, occurring in 20% of patients (n = 10) treated with oral semaglutide and 22% (n = 12) of patients treated with injectable semaglutide. Overall, 14% (n = 7) of patients taking oral semaglutide and none taking the injectable form complained of excessive belching. None of the participants discontinued the medication due to these side effects.

4. Discussion

Our study is the first direct comparison between the two semaglutide formulations in a real-world setting as add-on therapy to ongoing antihyperglycemic treatment in patients with inadequately controlled type 2 diabetes who had not previously received GLP-1 RA. Both formulations of semaglutide have been shown to be nearly equally effective in achieving HbA1c reduction (IS −1.1% vs. OS −1.4%) and weight loss (IS −6.5 kg vs. OS −5.9 kg).

Across the SUSTAIN program, once-weekly subcutaneous semaglutide 1.0 mg reduced HbA1c by 1.5–1.8% after 30–56 weeks, while once-daily oral semaglutide 14 mg reduced HbA1c by 1.0–1.4% across the PIONEER program [19,20]. In addition, subcutaneous semaglutide reduced body weight by 4.5 kg to 6.5 kg, significantly more than all active comparators tested, while oral semaglutide reduced body weight more than sitagliptin and liraglutide and to a similar extent as empagliflozin, namely between 2.6 kg and 4.4 kg. In a clinical trial conducted by Gibbons et al., people with a BMI of 20–38 kg/m^2 had less food cravings, had greater control over their diet, and consumed less food at each meal of the day with oral formulation of semaglutide versus the placebo [18]. Overall, after 12 weeks of treatment, the mean body weight decreased by 2.7 kg with oral semaglutide and 0.1 kg with placebo, mostly attributable to body fat mass loss [18].

Our results suggest that the antihyperglycemic potential of oral semaglutide in a real-world setting is consistent with that demonstrated in randomized clinical trials. However, the potential for weight reduction was more pronounced than in the PIONEER program. On the other hand, the HbA1c reduction achieved with the injectable form was slightly weaker than expected, but with body weight loss consistent with that in the SUSTAIN program. Moreover, the safety profile of the two formulations was similar. As commonly observed with GLP-1 Ras, the most common adverse side effect was nausea, which was generally mild to moderate and transient. Excessive belching was reported by 14% of patients taking oral semaglutide and by none of the patients taking the injectable form.

Given the generally similar efficacy and safety profiles of the two formulations, further considerations may need to be made in selecting the most appropriate formulation. Many patients are reluctant to initiate treatment with injectable medications due to fear of pain during injection and a sense of failure related to disease progression. A possible disadvantage of taking semaglutide orally is that the tablet must be taken on an empty stomach 30 min before a meal, drink, or taking other medications to ensure unimpeded absorption [17]. On the other hand, for injectable semaglutide, it does not matter whether food or liquid has been consumed before or after the injection. Therefore, selection of the most appropriate formulation needs to be made on an individual basis to best suit the patient's preferences and needs.

Our study suggests that semaglutide offers the benefits of a highly effective GLP-1 RA in both injectable and oral formulations. However, since this is a single-center retrospective observational study, the findings should be interpreted accordingly. It was conducted on a relatively small sample of respondents. Furthermore, due to the study design, the researchers had no control over exposures and interventions or absolute medication adherence. Likewise, there is the possibility of various confounding effects, such as background therapy and comorbidities. Nonetheless, our results have shown that orally administered semaglutide may be as effective an option for improving glycemic target attainment and supporting weight loss in adults with T2D as the injectable formulation, particularly in patients who are reluctant to take injectable medications.

5. Conclusions

In a real-world setting, oral semaglutide as an add-on therapy to ongoing antihyperglycemic treatment in patients with inadequately controlled type 2 diabetes who had not previously received GLP-1 RA demonstrated the same effectiveness as injectable semaglutide in terms of glycemic control and weight loss after 6 months of treatment. Considering the almost equal effect, the oral formulation of semaglutide could make it easier for patients to use since there is no injection burden.

Author Contributions: S.K. and A.B.—conception and design, data acquisition and analysis, review and editing; I.B.—data acquisition; N.M.—original draft preparation; D.R.—supervision. All authors have read and agreed to the published version of the manuscript.

Funding: This research received no external funding.

Institutional Review Board Statement: The study was conducted according to the guidelines of the Declaration of Helsinki and approved by the Institutional Review Board of Clinical Hospital Center Rijeka (No: 003-05/20-1/54).

Informed Consent Statement: Informed consent was obtained from all subjects involved in the study.

Data Availability Statement: The raw data supporting the conclusions of this article will be made available by the authors on request.

Conflicts of Interest: Sanja Klobučar is the Vice President of the Croatian Society for Diabetes and Metabolic Disorders of the Croatian Medical Association and the Vice President of the Croatian Society for Obesity of the Croatian Medical Association. She serves as an Executive Committee member of the Croatian Endocrine Society. She has served as the principal investigator or co-investigator in clinical trials of Eli Lilly, MSD, Novo Nordisk, and Sanofi Aventis. She has received honoraria for speaking or advisory board engagements and consulting fees from Abbott, AstraZeneca, Boehringer Ingelheim, Eli Lilly, Lifescan—Johnson & Johnson, Novartis, Novo Nordisk, MSD, Merck Sharp & Dohme, Mylan, Pliva, and Sanofi Aventis. Dario Raheli'c is the Director of the Vuk Vrhovac University Clinic for Diabetes, Endocrinology, and Metabolic Diseases at Merkur University Hospital, Zagreb, Croatia. He is the President of the Croatian Society for Diabetes and Metabolic Disorders of the Croatian Medical Association. He serves as an Executive Committee member of the Croatian Endocrine Society, Croatian Society for Obesity, and Croatian Society for Endocrine Oncology. He was a Board Member and Secretary of IDF Europe, and the Chair of the IDF Young Leaders in Diabetes (YLD) Program. He has served as an Executive Committee member of the Diabetes and Nutrition Study Group of the European Association for the Study of Diabetes (EASD), and currently, he serves as an Executive Committee member of the Diabetes and Cardiovascular Disease Study Group of EASD. He has served as a principal investigator or co-investigator in clinical trials for AstraZeneca, Eli Lilly, MSD, Novo Nordisk, Sanofi Aventis, Solvay, and Trophos. He has received honoraria for speaking or advisory board engagements and consulting fees from Abbott, Amgen, AstraZeneca, Bauerfeund, Bayer, Boehringer Ingelheim, Eli Lilly, Lifescan—Johnson & Johnson, Novartis, Novo Nordisk, MSD, Mylan, Pfizer, Pliva, Roche, Salvus, Sanofi Aventis, and Takeda. The other authors declare no conflicts of interest.

References

1. Sun, H.; Saeedi, P.; Karuranga, S.; Pinkepank, M.; Ogurtsova, K.; Duncan, B.B.; Stein, C.; Basit, A.; Chan, J.C.N.; Mbanya, J.C.; et al. IDF Diabetes Atlas: Global, regional and country-level diabetes prevalence estimates for 2021 and projections for 2045. *Diabetes Res. Clin. Pract.* **2022**, *183*, 109119. [CrossRef] [PubMed]
2. Einarson, T.R.; Acs, A.; Ludwig, C.; Panton, U.H. Prevalence of cardiovascular disease in type 2 diabetes: A systematic literature review of scientific evidence from across the world in 2007–2017. *Cardiovasc. Diabetol.* **2018**, *17*, 83. [CrossRef] [PubMed]
3. American Diabetes Association. Economic Costs of Diabetes in the US in 2017. *Diabetes Care* **2018**, *41*, 917–928. [CrossRef]
4. King, D.E.; Mainous, A.G., III; Buchanan, T.A.; Pearson, W.S. C-Reactive Protein and Glycemic Control in Adults with Diabetes. *Diabetes Care* **2003**, *26*, 1535–1539. [CrossRef]
5. McGurnaghan, S.; Blackbourn, L.A.K.; Mocevic, E.; Haagen Panton, U.; McCrimmon, R.J.; Sattar, N.; Wild, S.; Colhoun, H.M. Cardiovascular Disease Prevalence and Risk Factor Prevalence in Type 2 Diabetes: A Contemporary Analysis. *Diabet. Med.* **2019**, *36*, 718–725. [CrossRef] [PubMed]
6. CDC. Coronavirus Disease 2019. Available online: https://www.cdc.gov/chronicdisease/ (accessed on 5 April 2023).
7. American Heart Association. Available online: https://www.heart.org/ (accessed on 20 March 2023).

8. Grant, P.J.; Cosentino, F. The 2019 ESC Guidelines on Diabetes, Pre-Diabetes, and Cardiovascular Diseases Developed in Collaboration with the EASD: New Features and the 'Ten Commandments' of the 2019 Guidelines Are Discussed by Professor Peter J. Grant and Professor Francesco Cosentino, the Task Force Chairmen. *Eur. Heart J.* **2019**, *40*, 3215–3217. [CrossRef] [PubMed]
9. ElSayed, N.A.; Aleppo, G.; Aroda, V.R.; Bannuru, R.R.; Brown, F.M.; Bruemmer, D.; Collins, B.S.; Hilliard, M.E.; Isaacs, D.; Johnson, E.L.; et al. 8. Obesity and Weight Management for the Prevention and Treatment of Type 2 Diabetes: Standards of Care in Diabetes—2023. *Diabetes Care* **2023**, *46*, S128–S139. [CrossRef] [PubMed]
10. Narayan, K.M.V.; Boyle, J.P.; Thompson, T.J.; Gregg, E.W.; Williamson, D.F. Effect of BMI on Lifetime Risk for Diabetes in the U.S. *Diabetes Care* **2007**, *30*, 1562–1566. [CrossRef] [PubMed]
11. Sharma, A.; Verma, S. Mechanisms by Which Glucagon-Like-Peptide-1 Receptor Agonists and Sodium-Glucose Cotransporter-2 Inhibitors Reduce Cardiovascular Risk in Adults With Type 2 Diabetes Mellitus. *Can. J. Diabetes* **2020**, *44*, 93–102. [CrossRef] [PubMed]
12. Lyseng-Williamson, K.A. Glucagon-like Peptide-1 Receptor Agonists in Type-2 Diabetes: Their Uses and Differential Features. *Clin. Drug Investig.* **2019**, *39*, 805–819. [CrossRef]
13. Lin, D.S.-H.; Lee, J.-K.; Chen, W.-J. Major Adverse Cardiovascular and Limb Events in Patients with Diabetes Treated with GLP-1 Receptor Agonists vs DPP-4 Inhibitors. *Diabetologia* **2021**, *64*, 1949–1962. [CrossRef] [PubMed]
14. Buckley, S.T.; Bækdal, T.A.; Vegge, A.; Maarbjerg, S.J.; Pyke, C.; Ahnfelt-Rønne, J.; Madsen, K.G.; Schéele, S.G.; Alanentalo, T.; Kirk, R.K.; et al. Transcellular Stomach Absorption of a Derivatized Glucagon-like Peptide-1 Receptor Agonist. *Sci. Transl. Med.* **2018**, *10*, eaar7047. [CrossRef] [PubMed]
15. Andersen, A.; Knop, F.K.; Vilsbøll, T. A Pharmacological and Clinical Overview of Oral Semaglutide for the Treatment of Type 2 Diabetes. *Drugs* **2021**, *81*, 1003–1030. [CrossRef] [PubMed]
16. HIGHLIGHTS OF PRESCRIBING INFORMATION These Highlights Do Not Include All the Information Needed to Use RYBELSUS ® Safely and Effectively. See Full Prescribing Information for RYBELSUS. RYBELSUS (Semaglutide) Tablets, for Oral Use Initial U.S. Approval: 2017 WARNING: RISK OF THYROID C-CELL TUMORS See Full Prescribing Information for Complete Boxed Warning. Available online: https://www.accessdata.fda.gov/drugsatfda_docs/label/2019/213051s000lbl.pdf (accessed on 15 March 2023).
17. Rybelsus. Summary of Product Characteristics. Available online: https://www.ema.europa.eu/en/documents/productinformation/rybelsus-epar-product-information_en.pdf (accessed on 15 March 2023).
18. Gibbons, C.; Blundell, J.; Tetens Hoff, S.; Dahl, K.; Bauer, R.; Baekdal, T. Effects of Oral Semaglutide on Energy Intake, Food Preference, Appetite, Control of Eating and Body Weight in Subjects with Type 2 Diabetes. *Diabetes Obes. Metab.* **2021**, *23*, 581–588. [CrossRef] [PubMed]
19. Meier, J.J. Efficacy of Semaglutide in a Subcutaneous and an Oral Formulation. *Front. Endocrinol.* **2021**, *12*, 645617. [CrossRef] [PubMed]
20. Capehorn, M.S.; Catarig, A.-M.; Furberg, J.K.; Janez, A.; Price, H.C.; Tadayon, S.; Vergès, B.; Marre, M. Efficacy and Safety of Once-Weekly Semaglutide 1.0 Mg vs Once-Daily Liraglutide 1.2 Mg as Add-on to 1–3 Oral Antidiabetic Drugs in Subjects with Type 2 Diabetes (SUSTAIN 10). *Diabetes Metab.* **2020**, *46*, 100–109. [CrossRef] [PubMed]

Disclaimer/Publisher's Note: The statements, opinions and data contained in all publications are solely those of the individual author(s) and contributor(s) and not of MDPI and/or the editor(s). MDPI and/or the editor(s) disclaim responsibility for any injury to people or property resulting from any ideas, methods, instructions or products referred to in the content.

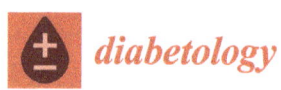 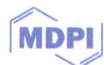

Article

Does the Efficacy of Semaglutide Treatment Differ between Low-Risk and High-Risk Subgroups of Patients with Type 2 Diabetes and Obesity Based on SCORE2, SCORE2-Diabetes, and ASCVD Calculations?

Martina Matovinović [1,*], Andrej Belančić [2,3], Juraj Jug [4], Filip Mustač [5,*], Maja Sirovica [6], Mihovil Santini [7], Anja Bošnjaković [8], Mario Lovrić [8,9] and Martina Lovrić Benčić [10,11]

1. Department of Internal Medicine, Division of Endocrinology, University Hospital Centre Zagreb, Croatian Referral Center for Obesity Treatment, Kišpatićeva 12, 10000 Zagreb, Croatia
2. Department of Clinical Pharmacology, Clinical Hospital Centre Rijeka, Krešimirova 42, 51000 Rijeka, Croatia; andrej.belancic@uniri.hr or a.belancic93@gmail.com
3. Department of Basic and Clinical Pharmacology with Toxicology, Faculty of Medicine, University of Rijeka, Braće Branchetta 20, 51000 Rijeka, Croatia
4. Health Center Zagreb—West, Department of Family Medicine, Prilaz Baruna Filipovića 11, 10000 Zagreb, Croatia; juraj2304@gmail.com
5. Department of Psychiatry and Psychological Medicine, University Hospital Centre Zagreb, Kišpatićeva 12, 10000 Zagreb, Croatia
6. Department of Anesthesiology, Resuscitation and Intensive Care Medicine and Pain Therapy, University Hospital Centre Zagreb, Kišpatićeva 12, 10000 Zagreb, Croatia; maja.sirovica@gmail.com
7. Department of Emergency, General Hospital Zadar, Bože Peričića 5, 23000 Zadar, Croatia; 023miho@gmail.com
8. Centre for Applied Bioanthropology, Institute for Anthropological Research, Ljudevita Gaja 32, 10000 Zagreb, Croatia; anja.bosnjakovic@inantro.hr (A.B.); mario.lovric@inantro.hr (M.L.)
9. Faculty of Electrical Engineering, Computer Science and Information Technology Osijek, Josip Juraj Strossmayer University of Osijek, Kneza Trpimira 2b, 31000 Zagreb, Croatia
10. Department of Cardiovascular Diseases, University Hospital Centre Zagreb, Kišpatićeva 12, 10000 Zagreb, Croatia; martina.lovric@zg.t-com.hr or miminamama@gmail.com
11. School of Medicine, University of Zagreb, Šalata 3, 10000 Zagreb, Croatia
* Correspondence: martina_10000@yahoo.com (M.M.); filip.mustac@gmail.com (F.M.)

Abstract: Background: Diabetes is the primary contributor to cardiovascular disease risk, and when combined with obesity, it further underscores the significance of cardiovascular risk assessment. Methods: A retrospective study of 64 patients with type 2 diabetes (T2D) and obesity on once-weekly subcutaneous semaglutide stratified by cardiovascular risk categories determined using the SCORE2/SCORE2-OP, SCORE2-Diabetes, and ASCVD score calculations. We compare the differences between groups (ASCVD: low + borderline + intermediate versus high-risk group; SCORE2/SCORE2-OP: low + moderate versus high + very high-risk group and SCORE2-Diabetes: low + moderate versus high + very high-risk group) in terms of change from baseline in body mass index (BMI) and HbA1c and weight loss outcomes. Results: Patients in the high-risk group, according to ASCVD risk score, had statistically better results in weight loss ≥ 3%, ≥5%, and ≥10% compared to ASCVD low + borderline + intermediate and without difference regarding HbA1c. According to SCORE2/SCORE2-OP, the high + very high-risk group had statistically better HbA1c and weight loss results but only for ≥5% versus the low + moderate risk group. Based on the score SCORE2-Diabetes, the high + very high-risk group had statistically significant better results in lowering HbA1c and weight loss but only for ≥5% versus the low + moderate risk group. Conclusions: To the best of our knowledge, this study represents the initial investigation linking glycemic control and weight reduction outcomes in individuals with T2D and obesity treated with once-weekly semaglutide stratified by cardiovascular risk categories determined using the SCORE2/SCORE2-OP, SCORE2-Diabetes and ASCVD score calculations.

Keywords: ASCVD risk score; SCORE2; SCORE2-diabetes; semaglutide; type 2 diabetes; obesity

Citation: Matovinović, M.; Belančić, A.; Jug, J.; Mustač, F.; Sirovica, M.; Santini, M.; Bošnjaković, A.; Lovrić, M.; Lovrić Benčić, M. Does the Efficacy of Semaglutide Treatment Differ between Low-Risk and High-Risk Subgroups of Patients with Type 2 Diabetes and Obesity Based on SCORE2, SCORE2-Diabetes, and ASCVD Calculations? *Diabetology* **2024**, *5*, 26–39. https://doi.org/10.3390/diabetology5010003

Academic Editor: Keiichiro Matoba

Received: 1 November 2023
Revised: 28 November 2023
Accepted: 2 January 2024
Published: 4 January 2024

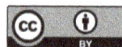

Copyright: © 2024 by the authors. Licensee MDPI, Basel, Switzerland. This article is an open access article distributed under the terms and conditions of the Creative Commons Attribution (CC BY) license (https:// creativecommons.org/licenses/by/ 4.0/).

1. Introduction

Type 2 diabetes and obesity are global health concerns with increasing prevalence worldwide. Both conditions are associated with a myriad of complications, including cardiovascular diseases, which contribute significantly to morbidity and mortality [1]. This strong association between diabetes and cardiovascular disease is widely acknowledged, with diabetes increasing the risk of coronary artery disease by a factor of two to four [2]. Therefore, it is essential for both healthcare providers and patients with type 2 diabetes (T2D) to undergo a risk assessment using tools such as the ASCVD (atherosclerotic cardiovascular disease) calculator [3] and SCORE2 (Systematic Coronary Risk Evaluation) [4]. The ASCVD Risk estimation is a universally accepted set of guidelines designed to forecast the likelihood of atherosclerotic cardiovascular disease (ASCVD) in individuals. It is employed for patients considered to be at risk of ASCVD. This estimation encompasses several key factors, and essential elements of the risk evaluation include the following: age (validated exclusively for patients aged 40 to 79), gender, total cholesterol levels, HDL cholesterol levels, systolic blood pressure, blood pressure treatment status (yes or no), presence of diabetes mellitus (yes or no), and current smoking status (yes or no) [5]. SCORE2 represents an updated algorithm specifically tailored for European populations, aiming to forecast the 10-year risk of initial cardiovascular disease (CVD) occurrence. This advancement enhances the ability to identify individuals at a heightened risk of developing CVD throughout Europe. The algorithm's development involved the analysis of data from a substantial pool of over 12.5 million individuals across numerous countries. In comparison to SCORE, SCORE2 offers several advantages, as follows: (1) it provides improved estimates of the overall CVD burden, particularly for younger individuals, and demonstrates superior risk discrimination; (2) it factors in the impact of competing risks, including non-CVD-related deaths; (3) it categorizes Europe into four distinct regions with varying CVD risk levels. However, it is important to note that this model has potential limitations. The risk prediction models were primarily derived from 45 cohorts, mainly in European regions and populations with low to moderate CVD risk. Additionally, the model assumes that the relative risks observed in the derivation dataset are applicable across diverse populations [4,6]. The SCORE2-OP risk prediction algorithm serves the purpose of assessing the risk of incident cardiovascular events in individuals aged 70 years or older residing in four distinct geographical risk regions. Most of the existing 10-year cardiovascular disease (CVD) risk prediction models exhibit limited effectiveness when applied to older individuals. SCORE2-OP overcomes this limitation by amalgamating data from three previously established CVD risk algorithms designed specifically for older populations. This model facilitates the estimation of combined outcomes, encompassing both fatal and non-fatal CVD events, and it also enables the calculation of the absolute reduction in CVD risk upon reaching treatment targets for blood pressure and LDL cholesterol. Nonetheless, it is important to acknowledge some potential constraints of this model. Firstly, its development relied on data from a cohort study in a region with low CVD risk. Secondly, certain predictors related to comorbidities or frailty, which might be significant factors in older individuals' CVD risk, were omitted from SCORE2-OP due to data availability constraints [7]. To effectively manage individuals who have both T2D and obesity, it is vital to evaluate each patient's cardiovascular risk. Subsequently, a treatment plan should be developed, and ongoing patient monitoring should be established. Patient monitoring can potentially improve early detection of cardiovascular risk in T2D patients, leading to improved patient outcomes and reduced healthcare costs [8]. Atherosclerotic cardiovascular disease stands as the primary contributor to illness and death among individuals with diabetes, leading to an estimated annual expenditure of USD 37.3 billion on diabetes-related cardiovascular care. On average, individuals with a confirmed diabetes diagnosis incur medical costs that are approximately 2.3 times greater than their expenses if they do not have diabetes [9–11]. The American Heart Association has advocated for the adoption of preventive measures, emphasizing the importance of addressing obesity in order to alleviate the impact of heart disease [9,10]. Presently, the American Diabetes Association (ADA) guidelines recommend using the ASCVD Risk Estimator Plus tool to assess the initial 10-year cardiovascular risk of experiencing ASCVD events [3,10].

Recently, a newly developed algorithm called SCORE2-diabetes underwent calibration and validation in four European regions to forecast the 10-year risk of CVD in individuals with T2D. This innovative tool incorporates diabetes-specific variables, including the age at diabetes diagnosis, glycated hemoglobin (HbA1c), and the estimated glomerular filtration rate (eGFR), in addition to traditional risk factors [12]. The validation of SCORE2-Diabetes in four distinct European countries, each representing diverse risk regions. The validation of SCORE2-Diabetes across four European countries (Croatia, Malta, Spain, and Sweden) from different risk regions demonstrated the model's precision in forecasting the cardiovascular disease risk linked with type 2 diabetes, both on an individual and population-wide basis [12].

As a GLP-1 receptor agonist, semaglutide enhances the efficiency of GLP-1 through diverse mechanisms, including enhanced glucose-dependent insulin secretion, inhibition of glucagon release, and suppressed hepatic gluconeogenesis [13]. As a result of these multiple effects, semaglutide contributes to decreased levels of fasting and postprandial glycemia, along with a reduction in food energy intake and delay in gastric, ultimately leading to weight loss [13].

Therefore, lowering both HbA1c levels and body weight without the risk of hypoglycemia gives it a distinct status in the treatment of individuals with obesity and type 2 diabetes [14].

Semaglutide, an FDA and EMA-approved GLP-1 receptor agonist for managing type 2 diabetes, has demonstrated statistically significant reductions in cardiovascular events [13]. Additionally, semaglutide was registered with the same regulatory authorities but at a higher dose of 2.4 mg once weekly subcutaneously for the treatment of obesity as an addition to behavioral therapy [15–17].

Existing models for predicting CVD risk in primary prevention settings may have notable limitations, especially when applied to patients with both T2D and obesity. This study aims to ascertain whether there are variations in the effectiveness of semaglutide treatment in terms of glycemic control and weight loss between subgroups of low-risk and high-risk patients with type 2 diabetes and obesity, determined through ASCVD score, SCORE 2/SCORE2-OP, and SCORE2-Diabetes calculations.

2. Patients and Methods

This was a retrospective study of patients with T2D and obesity who were treated using an individual approach in ambulatory in University Hospital Centre Zagreb at Department of Endocrinology. This study analyzed patients receiving once-weekly subcutaneous semaglutide (Ozempic®) for glycemia regulation. Patients who reached a semaglutide dose of ≥ 0.5 mg (before ambulatory control endpoint assessment at 6–8 months post introduction) and had all the variables needed for SCORE2/SCORE2-OP, SCORE2-Diabetes, and ASCVD risk calculation were included in our study [methodology and principle extensively presented in Refs. [3,6].

All relevant demographic (age, gender, and race) and clinical [height, body weight (BW), body mass index (BMI), HbA1c, fasting glucose, presence of comorbidities (arterial hypertension, dyslipidemia, and hypothyroidism), as well as other variables needed for SCORE2/SCORE2-OP, SCORE2-Diabetes and ASCVD risk calculation (e.g., systolic blood pressure, total cholesterol and HDL cholesterol, smoking status, data on using antihypertensives and statins in chronic pharmacotherapy, duration of diabetes, eGFR)] were collected.

The standard principles of T2D and obesity care (assessments and follow-up, e.g., methodology and principles and cut-offs for measurements for all studied anthropometric and biochemical parameters as well for blood pressure measurement) within the Croatian Referral Center for Obesity Treatment (which is also EASO collaborating center for obesity management), which are the same methodology principles applied here, were recently extensively presented and published elsewhere [18].

SCORE2/SCORE-OP, SCORE2-Diabetes and ASCVD cardiovascular risk categories were calculated for each patient as per standardized and validated principles published by the European Society of Cardiology [extensively presented in Refs. [3,6,12].

Patients were divided into SCORE2/SCORE2-OP low + moderate (SCORE2 group 1) and SCORE2/SCORE2-OP high + very high-risk (SCORE2 group 2) groups, SCORE2-Diabetes low + moderate (SCORE2-Diabetes group 1) and SCORE2-Diabetes high + very high-risk (SCORE2-Diabetes group 2), as well as ASCVD low + borderline + intermediate (ASCVD group 1) and ASCVD high-risk (ASCVD group 2) groups in order to compare the results of semaglutide weight loss- and glycemia regulation-wise, depending on the baseline cardiovascular risk as a potential therapy effectiveness predictor.

Studied endpoints were changes in body weight ($\triangle$BMI, and $\triangle$BW $\geq$ 3%, $\triangle$BW $\geq$ 5%, and $\triangle$BW $\geq$ 10% percentage of patients) and glycemia ($\triangle$HbA1c) at the ambulatory check-up 6–8 months after the initiation of the once-weekly subcutaneous semaglutide (Ozempic®).

The study was approved by the local Ethics Committee of the University Hospital Centre Zagreb, Croatia. Bearing in mind the retrospective nature of the study and its design, as well as the fact that the used data had been anonymized and already recorded, a waiver of informed consent was approved (Permit class: 8.1-18/161-2, No. 02/21 AG). Overall, the study was conducted in accordance with the Declaration of Helsinki.

Statistical Analysis

Statistical analysis was performed using Microsoft Excel version 2311 (Microsoft Office, Redmond, WA, USA) and MedCalc v14.8.1 (MedCalc Software bvba, Ostend, Belgium) and Python (v3.9.10). Absolute and relative frequencies, measures of central tendency alongside measures of spread, were used to present the data. The Kolmogorov–Smirnov test was used to assess the normality of distribution. Mann–Whitney test was used to compare the differences between groups (ASCVD: low + borderline + intermediate versus high-risk group; SCORE2: low + moderate versus high + very high-risk group, and SCORE2-Diabetes: low + moderate versus high + very high-risk group) in terms of change from baseline in BMI and HbA1c. Furthermore, to compare the differences (frequencies of patients) in other weight loss outcomes ($\triangle$BW $\geq$ 3%, $\triangle$BW $\geq$ 5%, and $\triangle$BW $\geq$ 10%), a χ2-test was used. All statistical tests were two-tailed and with a 95% CI. Overall, the criterion for statistical significance was set at $p < 0.05$.

3. Results

Overall, 64 patients [60.9% female; median age 57.5 (41–81) yr.] on once-weekly subcutaneous semaglutide meet our enrolment criteria. The vast majority of patients were severely obese and had a high cardiovascular risk (Table 1).

Comparison between subgroups (SCORE2 low + moderate vs. SCORE2 high + very high-risk group; SCORE2-Diabetes low + medium vs. SCORE2-Diabetes high + very high-risk group, and ASCVD low + borderline + intermediate vs. ASCVD high-risk group, with Mann–Whitney test) in terms of baseline BW, BMI, and HbA1c revealed the following: 131.1 $\pm$ 31.2 kg vs. 114.8 $\pm$ 23.6 kg (p = 0.064); 132.3 $\pm$ 30.4 vs. 119.1 $\pm$ 24.6 kg (p = 0.148), and 123.5 $\pm$ 28.7 kg vs. 113.9 $\pm$ 23.7 kg (p = 0.290); 46.6 $\pm$ 10.6 kg/m^2 vs. 40.4 $\pm$ 6.4 kg/m^2 (p = 0.017), 46.9 $\pm$ 10.9 vs. 41.7 $\pm$ 6.5 kg/m^2 (p = 0.101), and 43.6 $\pm$ 8.9 kg/m^2 vs. 40.2 $\pm$ 7.4 kg/m^2 (p = 0.097); 6.7 $\pm$ 1.0% vs. 7.5 $\pm$ 1.3% (p = 0.018), 6.6 $\pm$ 0.9% vs. 7.4 $\pm$ 1.4% (p = 0.022), and 6.9 $\pm$ 1.2% vs. 7.8 $\pm$ 1.2% (p = 0.003), respectively.

Table 1. Demographic and baseline clinical characteristics of our T2D cohort (N = 64) using subcutaneous semaglutide once-weekly.

Gender distribution (%, N of female patients)		60.9%, 39
Age (Median, Min-Max, yr.)		57.5 (41–81)
Height (X ± SD, cm)		168.1 ± 10.1
Weight (X ± SD, kg)		120.4 ± 27.3
BMI (X ± SD, kg/m^2)		42.5 ± 8.5
BMI category distribution (%, N)	BMI < 25 kg/m^2	0%, 0
	Overweight	0%, 0
	Obesity class I	14.1%, 9
	Obesity class II	31.3%, 20
	Obesity class III	54.7%, 35
Comorbidities (%, N)	Arterial hypertension	79.7%, 51
	Dyslipidemia	84.4%, 54
	Hypothyroidism [1]	17.2%, 11
HbA1c (X ± SD, %)		7.2 ± 1.3
Fasting glucose (X ± SD, mmol/L)		8.6 ± 2.2
Semaglutide dose achieved (%, N)	0.5 mg	60.9%, 39
	1 mg	39.1%, 25
SCORE2 distribution (%, N)	Low	0%, 0
	Moderate	34.4%, 22
	High	43.7%, 28
	Very high	21.9%, 14
SCORE2-Diabetes distribution (%, N) [2]	Low	10.5%, 6
	Moderate	22.8%, 13
	High	42.1%, 24
	Very high	24.6%, 14
ASCVD distribution (%, N)	Low	15.6%, 10
	Borderline	14.1%, 9
	Intermediate	37.5%, 24
	High	32.8%, 21

[1] All patients were euthyroid during the study follow-up period, [2] Sample size = 57 patients.

Results of the Statistical Analysis

SCORE 2 high + very high-risk group had statistically better results in terms of △BMI (-2.4 ± 2.1 kg/m^2 vs. -1.3 ± 1.5 kg/m^2, $p = 0.045$; Figure 1) and △HbA1c (-0.9 ± 1.2% vs. -0.2 ± 0.9%, $p = 0.013$; Figure 2) as well as the frequency of patients who achieved △BW ≥ 5% (61.9% vs. 22.7%, $X^2 = 8.744$, $p = 0.003$), when compared to SCORE2 low + medium group. Not statistically significant differences between groups were revealed in terms of △BW ≥ 3% (73.8% vs. 54.5%, $X^2 = 2.400$, $p = 0.121$) and △BW ≥ 10% (21.4% vs. 4.5%, $X^2 = 3.084$, $p = 0.079$) frequencies.

SCORE2-Diabetes high + very high (N = 38) risk group, when compared to SCORE2-Diabetes low + medium (N = 19), had statistically better results in terms of △BMI (-2.4 ± 2.0 kg/m^2 vs. -1.1 ± 1.6 kg/m^2, $p = 0.039$; Figure 3), △BW ≥ 5% (57.9% vs. 21.0%, $X^2 = 6.831$, $p = 0.009$), and △HbA1c (-0.9 ± 1.2% vs. -0.2 ± 0.9%, $p = 0.028$; Figure 4). However, no statistically significant difference was found in terms of △BW ≥ 3%

(73.7% vs. 47.4%, $X^2 = 3.780$, $p = 0.052$) and $\triangle BW \geq 10\%$ (18.4% vs. 5.3%, $X^2 = 1.770$, $p = 0.183$).

The ASCVD high (N = 21) risk group had statistically better results in terms of all studied anthropometric/weight loss endpoints compared to ASCVD low + borderline + intermediate risk group (N = 43): $\triangle BMI$ (-2.8 ± 1.9 kg/m^2 vs. -1.7 ± 1.9 kg/m^2, $p = 0.030$; Figure 5), and $\triangle BW \geq 3\%$ (85.7% vs. 58.1%, $X^2 = 4.797$, $p = 0.028$), $\triangle BW \geq 5\%$ (71.4% vs. 37.2%, $X^2 = 6.504$, $p = 0.011$), and $\triangle BW \geq 10\%$ (28.6% vs. 9.3%, $X^2 = 3.923$, $p = 0.048$) frequencies. No difference was found regarding $\triangle HbA1c$ ($-1.2 \pm 1.1\%$ vs. $-0.4 \pm 1.1\%$, $p = 0.591$; Figure 6).

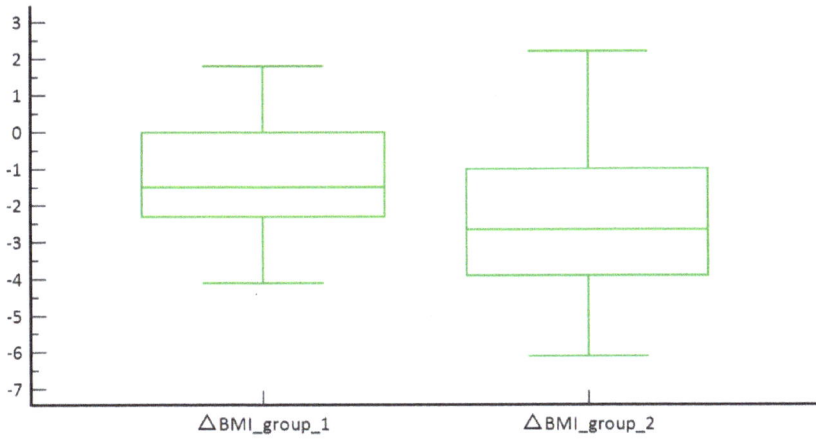

Figure 1. Comparison between SCORE2 low + medium (below SCORE2 group 1) vs. SCORE 2 high + very high-risk (above SCORE2 group 2) groups in terms of $\triangle BMI$.

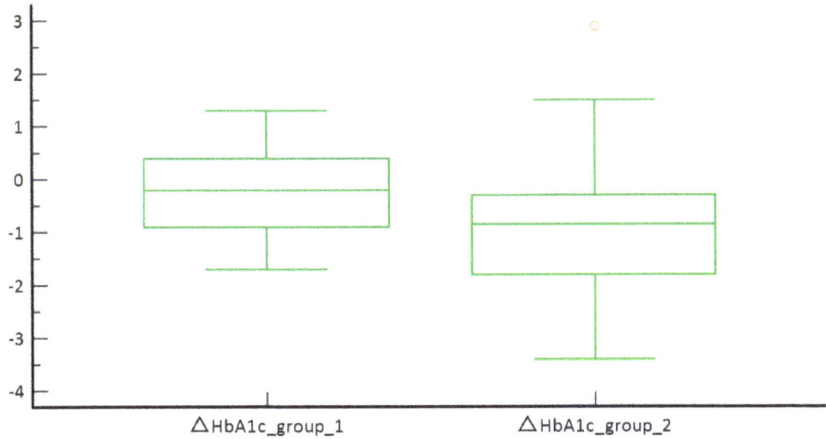

Figure 2. Comparison between SCORE2-Diabetes low + medium (above SCORE2-Diabetes group 1) vs. SCORE2-Diabetes high + very high risk (below SCORE2-Diabetes group 2) groups in terms of $\triangle BMI$.

Additionally, the use of other medication was inspected prior to semaglutide therapy.

Patients previously treated with SGLT2 inhibitors (N = 13) demonstrated a less pronounced reduction in BMI, with a mean change of -1.06 ± 2.09 kg/m^2, compared to a mean reduction of -2.28 ± 1.85 kg/m^2 in the untreated group (N = 51). This difference was statistically significant (U-value: 458.5, $p = 0.017353$), indicating a lesser degree of BMI reduction in the SGLT2 inhibitor-treated group (Figure 7).

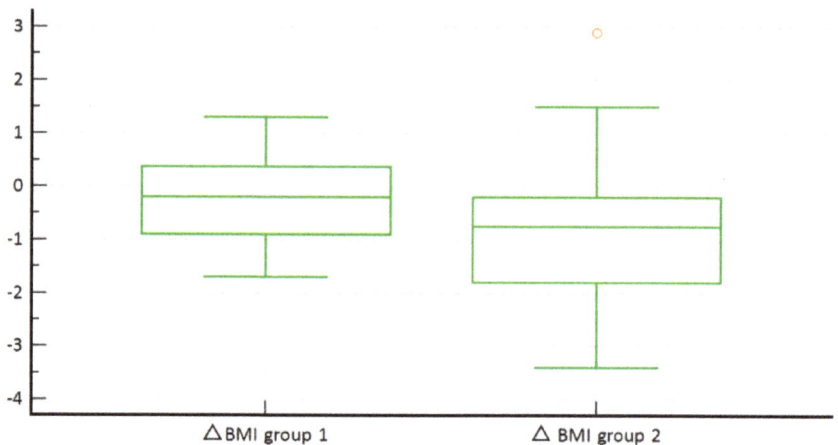

Figure 3. Comparison between SCORE2-Diabetes low + medium (above SCORE2-Diabetes group 1) vs. SCORE2-Diabetes high + very high-risk (below SCORE2-Diabetes group 2) groups in terms of △BMI.

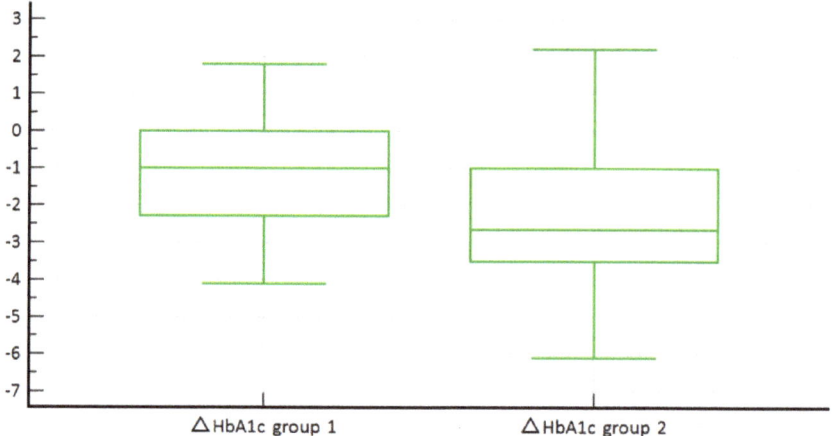

Figure 4. Comparison between SCORE2-Diabetes low + medium (above SCORE2-Diabetes group 1) vs. SCORE2-Diabetes high + very high-risk (below SCORE2-Diabetes group 2) groups in terms of △HbA1c.

In the comparison of delta HbA1c% levels, the group treated with SGLT2 inhibitors (N = 13) showed a mean reduction of $-0.41 \pm 1.34\%$, which was less than the $-0.72 \pm 1.09\%$ observed in the untreated group (N = 51). The statistical analysis yielded a U-value of 416.5 and a p-value of 0.079177, suggesting a trend towards a lesser reduction in HbA1c% among the SGLT2 inhibitor-treated patients, although this did not reach conventional levels of statistical significance (Figure 7).

Figure 8 shows that there is no significant difference in the intake of SGLT-2 inhibitors, concerning age, BMI, weight or the three scores. A Mann–Whitney U test confirmed this.

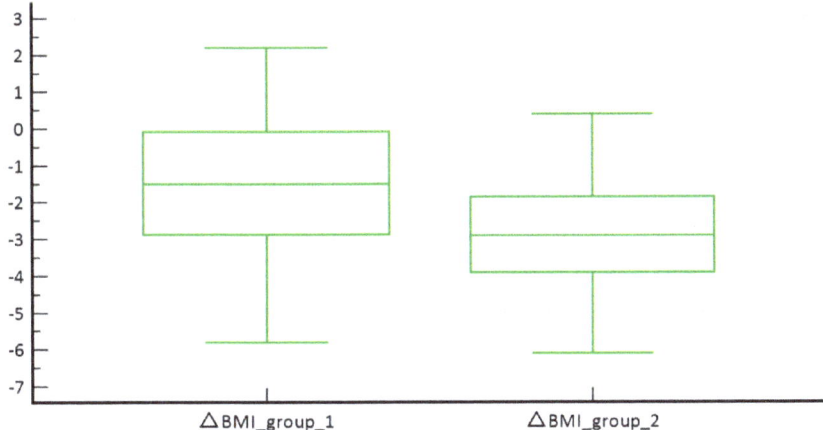

Figure 5. Comparison between ASCVD low + borderline + intermediate (above SCORE2 group 1) vs. ASCVD high risk (below SCORE2 group 2) groups in terms of △BMI.

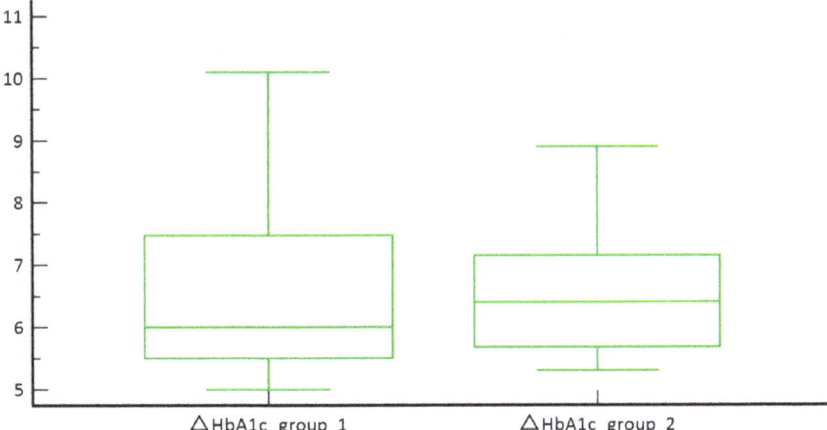

Figure 6. Comparison between ASCVD low + borderline + intermediate (below SCORE2 group 1) vs. ASCVD high risk (above SCORE2 group 2) groups in terms of △HbA1c.

For patients treated with other GLP-1 agonists (N = 18), the mean reduction in BMI was -1.29 ± 1.82 kg/m^2, compared to a more substantial mean reduction of -2.33 ± 1.93 kg/m^2 in the non-treated group (N = 46). This difference was statistically significant (U-value: 567.0, p = 0.011361), indicating a greater reduction in BMI among patients not treated with GLP-1 agonists.

Regarding the change in HbA1c% levels, patients treated with other GLP-1 agonists (N = 18) experienced a mean reduction of -0.41 ± 1.37%, in contrast to a mean reduction of -0.76 ± 1.03% in the non-treated group (N = 46). The statistical analysis showed a U-value of 518.5 and a p-value of 0.060143, indicating a trend towards a lesser reduction in HbA1c% in the GLP-1 agonist-treated group, though not reaching a level of statistical significance.

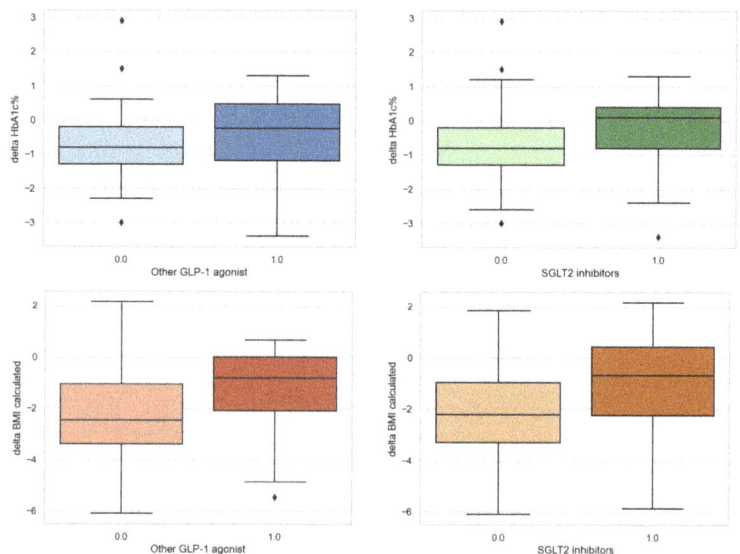

Figure 7. Comparison between patient who took Other GLP-1 agonists (**left** side) and SGL2 inhibitors (**right** side) groups in terms of △HbA1c (**top**) and △BMI (**bottom**).

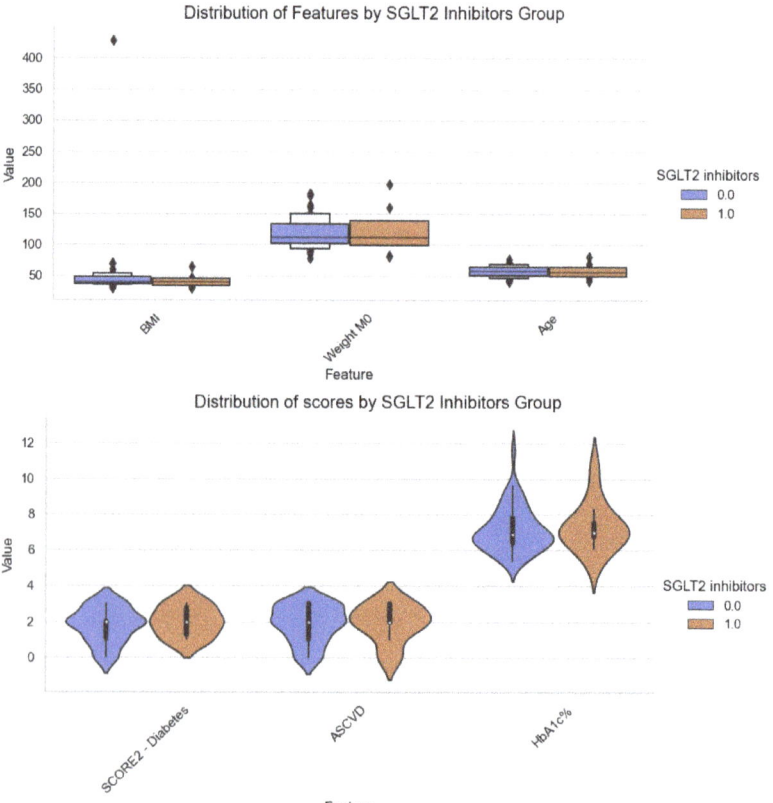

Figure 8. Differences in age and anthropometry in the groups of patients on SGLT2 inhibitors (1) and those who are not (0) in the upper figure, while the lower figure shows differences in the score.

4. Discussion

Mitigating cardiovascular risk holds significant importance in lowering morbidity rates among individuals with diabetes. This significance is amplified in patients who are concurrently dealing with both diabetes and obesity.

Selecting medications that effectively lower glucose levels, promote weight loss, and enhance cardiovascular outcomes is crucial for individuals dealing with both type 2 diabetes and obesity. The central message is that both categories of medications, including GLP-1 receptor agonists and SGLT2 inhibitors, have demonstrated their effectiveness in "proven cardiovascular efficacy". Semaglutide is one of the medications that showed these characteristics [19]. Noteworthy, obesity can double CVD risk in all patients with type 2 diabetes [20].

The SCORE 2/SCORE 2- OP high and very high-risk group showed statistically significant improvements in terms of reducing BMI and HbA1c levels, as well as a higher proportion of patients achieving weight loss $\geq$ 5% compared to the SCORE 2 low and moderate-risk group. There were not statistically significant differences between the two groups in terms of weight loss $\geq$ 3% and weight loss $\geq$ 10% achievement rates.

In the SUSTAIN-6 study, in patients with type 2 diabetes and with established cardiovascular disease, the rate of cardiovascular death, nonfatal myocardial infarction, or nonfatal stroke was shown to be significantly lower among patients receiving semaglutide than among those receiving placebo [13]. In this study, by week 104, patients treated with semaglutide experienced notable improvements when compared to those receiving a placebo. Specifically, their average glycated hemoglobin levels decreased from 8.7% at the beginning of the study to 7.6% (for the group receiving 0.5 mg) and 7.3% (for the group receiving 1.0 mg). Additionally, the mean body weight of patients receiving semaglutide decreased from an initial 92.1 kg to 88.5 kg (for the 0.5 mg group) and 87.2 kg (for the 1.0 mg group) [13].

In our study, the average glycated hemoglobin levels of participants (for the 0.5 mg and 1 mg groups) decreased from 7.2% initially to 6.5%. Additionally, patients receiving semaglutide experienced a reduction in mean body weight from 120.4 kg to 113.8 kg and a decrease in BMI from 42.5 kg/m^2 to 40.4 kg/m^2. In comparison to the SUSTAIN-6 study lasting 104 weeks, our study, conducted over 26 to 34 weeks, showed lower baseline HbA1c but higher baseline body weight and BMI, with a smaller drop in HbA1c and a greater reduction in body weight and BMI. This preliminary comparison highlights the need for an extended study duration to draw more meaningful conclusions.

These outcomes can be elucidated by the previously established mechanisms of action of semaglutide on glucose, HbA1c, and body weight [13].

In these cardiovascular outcomes trials, patients treated with semaglutide exhibited a significant 26% reduction in the risk of the primary composite outcome when compared to those receiving a placebo [13]. This risk reduction was primarily driven by a significant 39% decrease in nonfatal stroke rates and a nonsignificant 26% decrease in nonfatal myocardial infarction, with no significant difference in cardiovascular death rates. These risk reductions were consistent across both doses of semaglutide [13]. The SUSTAIN-6 and PIONEER-6 studies demonstrate the positive impact of semaglutide on reducing cardiovascular risk and post hoc analysis revealed approximately a 24% reduction in cardiovascular adverse events compared to the placebo [21].

Both the 0.5 mg and 1.0 mg doses of semaglutide demonstrate significant enhancements in glycemic management and body weight reduction in individuals with type 2 diabetes vs. comparators, irrespective of whether they are concurrently using other antidiabetic medications [22–24].

In our research, the exclusion criterion was a history of established CVD, which includes previous cardiovascular, cerebrovascular, or peripheral vascular diseases. However, we observed that those at high-risk (high and very high-risk group), as determined by the SCORE2/SCORE2-OP calculation, experienced more significant improvements in lowering HbA1c and reducing body weight in terms of a weight loss $\geq$ 5% versus the low-risk group (low and moderate). Nevertheless, our observations indicated that individuals in the high-risk category (comprising the high and very high-risk groups), as determined by the SCORE2/SCORE2-OP calculation, demonstrated more substantial enhancements in reducing HbA1c levels and weight loss $\geq 5\%$ compared to the low-risk group (consisting of the low and moderate-risk individuals). However, there were no discernible differences between groups regarding weight loss $\geq 3\%$ and $\geq 10\%$.

Patients with T2D on semaglutide in our study had a higher body mass index (BMI) and better glycemic control, reflected in lower average HbA1c levels, compared to patients in the SUSTAIN-6 study who received semaglutide.

The SCORE2-Diabetes algorithms were recently developed by extending SCORE2, using data from >220,000 patients with T2D with good external validation in >210.000 individuals from four countries, including Croatia [12]. However, similar outcomes in our study (weight loss $\geq 5\%$ and decreasing HbA1c) were in the risk group patients calculated via the SCORE2/SCORE2-OP and SCORE-Diabetes. It is possible that even more substantial changes could be observed if the observation period were extended.

Across all BMI subgroups, the individual SUSTAIN 1 to 5 trials [22–26] demonstrated that semaglutide resulted in significantly higher percentages of subjects achieving weight loss of $\geq 5\%$ and $\geq 10\%$ compared to the comparator groups, with a more pronounced effect observed with the 1.0 mg dose of semaglutide compared to the 0.5 mg dose. We demonstrated that individuals with type 2 diabetes and obesity who received once-weekly semaglutide treatment achieved significant weight loss ($\geq 3\%$, $\geq 5\%$, and $\geq 10\%$) in the high-risk group compared to the lower-risk group (comprising those with low, borderline, and intermediate risk) according to the ASCVD score although the initial BMI was lower in the high-risk group. However, there was no significant difference in terms of HbA1c reduction between these two groups.

Although other CVD risk prediction scores are recommended in patients with diabetes, the prediction of CVD via the SCORE system was significantly better than, for example, the UK Prospective Diabetes Study System [27]. The incorporation of diabetes as a categorical variable in the SCORE equation quadruples the CVD risk for diabetic women and doubles it for diabetic men. This equation does not consider the glycemic control or diabetes duration, which can under- or overestimate real CVD risk [28]. Because of its similarity, these limitations can also be applied to SCORE2 risk. Zhang et al. suggested that HbA1c values should be used in CVD risk assessment, especially in patients with HbA1c of 7–8% and low or moderate ASCVD score risk [29]. SCORE 2 and ASCVD risk are relatively new CVD risk assessment methods, and there are no scientific studies investigating the benefit of semaglutide in patients with lower or higher CVD risk assessed by them.

Patients with both type 2 diabetes and obesity, deemed at high risk based on the above score calculations, attained more favorable outcomes. These results can be partially attributed to our multidisciplinary approach comprising an endocrinologist-diabetologist, nutritionist, psychiatrist, psychologist, cardiologist, nephrologist, and neurologist for the treatment of individuals with obesity and/or T2D, aligning with the guidelines provided by the ADA guidelines [10,30]. Since patients with obesity and diabetes mellitus represent a great challenge, both in treatment, which does not only include pharmacotherapy but also a change in lifestyle is very important in order to achieve satisfactory results of treatment and control of the disease. Furthermore, the very use of any drug that is related to weight loss calls into question one's own active role in terms of whether something happens because of that medication or because of one's own behavior, which calls into question one's own motivation and requires a certain level of adaptation to the situation itself and direction of behavior. Mobile applications that can be used to quickly and easily monitor caloric intake and body weight and encourage exercise certainly play an interesting role [31,32]. Awareness of the problem of obesity can certainly be one of the focuses and therapeutic goals in psychotherapy, and an integrative approach that, together with an endocrinologist who deals specifically with obesity, together with a psychologist and a psychiatrist, can certainly help more than without psychological support [30,33]. An existing aspect among some of our patients includes pre-existing psychological conditions that can adversely affect individuals with diabetes in general. These conditions can influence factors such as motivation, self-care behaviors, glucose control, and medication adherence, all of which play a significant role in diabetes management. It is, therefore, important to pay attention to these psychological barriers as a vital step in enhancing diabetes care and addressing the individual challenges posed by this disease [34].

Equally, in today's world, there is mostly an insistence on instant solutions, fast diets that can quickly lose body weight, but most contemporary research claims that there is no universally successful diet, from the Mediterranean to intermittent fasting [35–38].

The analysis of medication use revealed that patients previously treated with SGLT2 inhibitors exhibited a significantly lesser reduction in BMI compared to those not treated with these inhibitors. However, the difference in HbA1c% reduction between the treated and untreated groups, although trending towards lesser reduction in the treated group, did not reach statistical significance. Similarly, patients treated with other GLP-1 agonists showed a lesser reduction in both BMI and HbA1c% compared to their untreated counterparts, with the difference in BMI being statistically significant. These findings suggest that prior treatment with SGLT2 inhibitors and other GLP-1 agonists may influence the effectiveness of interventions aimed at reducing BMI and HbA1c% levels.

5. Limitations

None of the scoring systems (ASCVD, SCORE2/SCORE-OP, and SCORE-Diabetes) incorporate BMI as an element within the cardiovascular risk assessment algorithm. In forthcoming research, it is recommended to involve a greater number of patients with diabetes and obesity class 2 and 3 for comparison with individuals of normal body weight or those who are overweight to see if there is a difference in the 10-year prediction of CVD according to BMI.

The sample size for this study is relatively small, so in the future, a larger sample size would enhance the study's robustness and generalizability. Additionally, in the future investigation, it would be preferable to ensure a more balanced representation among the stratified risk groups.

6. Conclusions

The effectiveness of semaglutide therapy in individuals with type 2 diabetes and obesity was confirmed in those categorized as high-risk according to ASCVD calculations, as well as according to SCORE/SCORE2-OP and SCORE-Diabetes assessments. Patients with higher risk experienced more substantial improvements in glycemic control, resulting in lower HbA1c levels and weight reduction, even though they initially had a lower BMI when they began treatment. Further research is necessary to expand the study population, encompassing individuals with both diabetes and obesity, as well as those without obesity who received weekly subcutaneous semaglutide. This research assessed the variations in treatment effectiveness between these groups based on their ASCVD, SCORE2/SCORE-OP, and SCORE2-Diabetes risk assessments.

Author Contributions: Conceptualization, M.M. and A.B. (Andrej Belančić); methodology, M.M. and A.B. (Andrej Belančić); software, A.B. (Anja Bošnjaković); validation, A.B. (Andrej Belančić) and M.M.; formal analysis, M.M. and A.B. (Andrej Belančić); investigation, M.M.; resources, M.M.; data curation, M.M., M.S. (Mihovil Santini), M.S. (Maja Sirovica) and A.B. (Andrej Belančić); writing—original draft preparation, M.M. and A.B. (Andrej Belančić); writing—review and editing, M.M., A.B. (Andrej Belančić), J.J. and F.M.; visualization, A.B. (Andrej Belančić), M.M. and M.L.; supervision, M.M., A.B. (Andrej Belančić) and M.L.B. All authors have read and agreed to the published version of the manuscript.

Funding: This research received no external funding.

Institutional Review Board Statement: The study was conducted in accordance with the Declaration of Helsinki, and approved by the Institutional Review Board (or Ethics Committee) of University Hospital Center Zagreb (Permit class: 8.1-18/161-2, No. 02/21 AG).

Informed Consent Statement: Informed consent was obtained from all subjects involved in the study.

Data Availability Statement: Data available upon reasonable request send to the corresponding author.

Acknowledgments: We thank all participants of the cohort. The graphical abstract was created with BioRender.com (accessed on 29 November 2023).

Conflicts of Interest: The authors declare no conflicts of interest.

References

1. World Health Organization Diabetes. Available online: https://www.who.int/health-topics/diabetes (accessed on 11 October 2023).
2. Yusuf, S.; Hawken, S.; Ounpuu, S.; Dans, T.; Avezum, A.; Lanas, F.; McQueen, M.; Budaj, A.; Pais, P.; Varigos, J.; et al. Effect of Potentially Modifiable Risk Factors Associated with Myocardial Infarction in 52 Countries (the INTERHEART Study): Case-Control Study. *Lancet Lond. Engl.* **2004**, *364*, 937–952. [CrossRef] [PubMed]
3. ASCVD Risk Estimator Plus. Available online: https://www.acc.org/Tools-and-Practice-Support/Mobile-Resources/Features/http://www.acc.org/Tools-and-Practice-Support/Mobile-Resources/Features/2013-Prevention-Guidelines-ASCVD-Risk-Estimator (accessed on 14 September 2023).
4. SCORE2 Working Group and ESC Cardiovascular Risk Collaboration. SCORE2 Risk Prediction Algorithms: New Models to Estimate 10-Year Risk of Cardiovascular Disease in Europe. *Eur. Heart J.* **2021**, *42*, 2439–2454. [CrossRef] [PubMed]
5. Goff, D.C.; Lloyd-Jones, D.M.; Bennett, G.; Coady, S.; D'Agostino, R.B.; Gibbons, R.; Greenland, P.; Lackland, D.T.; Levy, D.; O'Donnell, C.J.; et al. 2013 ACC/AHA Guideline on the Assessment of Cardiovascular Risk: A Report of the American College of Cardiology/American Heart Association Task Force on Practice Guidelines. *Circulation* **2014**, *129*, S49–S73. [CrossRef] [PubMed]
6. Conroy, R.M.; Pyörälä, K.; Fitzgerald, A.P.; Sans, S.; Menotti, A.; De Backer, G.; De Bacquer, D.; Ducimetière, P.; Jousilahti, P.; Keil, U.; et al. SCORE project group. Estimation of ten-year risk of fatal cardiovascular disease in Europe: The SCORE project. *Eur. Heart J.* **2003**, *24*, 987–1003. [CrossRef] [PubMed]
7. SCORE2-OP Working Group and ESC Cardiovascular Risk Collaboration. SCORE2-OP Risk Prediction Algorithms: Estimating Incident Cardiovascular Event Risk in Older Persons in Four Geographical Risk Regions. *Eur. Heart J.* **2021**, *42*, 2455–2467. [CrossRef] [PubMed]
8. Fox, C.S.; Golden, S.H.; Anderson, C.; Bray, G.A.; Burke, L.E.; de Boer, I.H.; Deedwania, P.; Eckel, R.H.; Ershow, A.G.; Fradkin, J.; et al. Update on Prevention of Cardiovascular Disease in Adults with Type 2 Diabetes Mellitus in Light of Recent Evidence: A Scientific Statement from the American Heart Association and the American Diabetes Association. *Diabetes Care* **2015**, *38*, 1777–1803. [CrossRef] [PubMed]
9. American Diabetes Association. Economic Costs of Diabetes in the U.S. in 2017. *Diabetes Care* **2018**, *41*, 917–928. [CrossRef]
10. ElSayed, N.A.; Aleppo, G.; Aroda, V.R.; Bannuru, R.R.; Brown, F.M.; Bruemmer, D.; Collins, B.S.; Hilliard, M.E.; Isaacs, D.; Johnson, E.L.; et al. Obesity and Weight Management for the Prevention and Treatment of Type 2 Diabetes: Standards of Care in Diabetes—2023. *Diabetes Care* **2023**, *46*, S128–S139. [CrossRef]
11. Colombi, A.M.; Wood, G.C. Obesity in the Workplace: Impact on Cardiovascular Disease, Cost, and Utilization of Care. *Am. Health Drug Benefits* **2011**, *4*, 271–278.
12. SCORE2-Diabetes Working Group and the ESC Cardiovascular Risk Collaboration; Pennells, L.; Kaptoge, S.; Østergaard, H.B.; Read, S.H.; Carinci, F.; Franch-Nadal, J.; Petitjean, C.; Taylor, O.; Hageman, S.H.J.; et al. SCORE2-Diabetes: 10-Year Cardiovascular Risk Estimation in Type 2 Diabetes in Europe. *Eur. Heart J.* **2023**, *44*, 2544–2556. [CrossRef]
13. Marso, S.P.; Bain, S.C.; Consoli, A.; Eliaschewitz, F.G.; Jódar, E.; Leiter, L.A.; Lingvay, I.; Rosenstock, J.; Seufert, J.; Warren, M.L.; et al. Semaglutide and Cardiovascular Outcomes in Patients with Type 2 Diabetes. *N. Engl. J. Med.* **2016**, *375*, 1834–1844. [CrossRef]
14. Mahapatra, M.K.; Karuppasamy, M.; Sahoo, B.M. Semaglutide, a Glucagon like Peptide-1 Receptor Agonist with Cardiovascular Benefits for Management of Type 2 Diabetes. *Rev. Endocr. Metab. Disord.* **2022**, *23*, 521–539. [CrossRef] [PubMed]
15. Wadden, T.A.; Bailey, T.S.; Billings, L.K.; Davies, M.; Frias, J.P.; Koroleva, A.; Lingvay, I.; O'Neil, P.M.; Rubino, D.M.; Skovgaard, D.; et al. Effect of Subcutaneous Semaglutide vs Placebo as an Adjunct to Intensive Behavioral Therapy on Body Weight in Adults with Overweight or Obesity: The STEP 3 Randomized Clinical Trial. *JAMA* **2021**, *325*, 1403–1413. [CrossRef] [PubMed]
16. FDA Approves Higher Semaglutide Dose for Obesity. Available online: https://diabetes.medicinematters.com/semaglutide/obesity/step-trials-fda-approves-semaglutide-dose-obesity/19231776 (accessed on 27 November 2023).
17. EMA Wegovy. Available online: https://www.ema.europa.eu/en/medicines/human/EPAR/wegovy (accessed on 27 November 2023).
18. Bažadona, D.; Matovinović, M.; Krbot Skorić, M.; Grbavac, H.; Belančić, A.; Malojčić, B. The Interconnection between Carotid Intima–Media Thickness and Obesity: Anthropometric, Clinical and Biochemical Correlations. *Medicina* **2023**, *59*, 1512. [CrossRef] [PubMed]

19. Marx, N.; Federici, M.; Schütt, K.; Müller-Wieland, D.; Ajjan, R.A.; Antunes, M.J.; Christodorescu, R.M.; Crawford, C.; Di Angelantonio, E.; Eliasson, B.; et al. 2023 ESC Guidelines for the Management of Cardiovascular Disease in Patients with Diabetes: Developed by the Task Force on the Management of Cardiovascular Disease in Patients with Diabetes of the European Society of Cardiology (ESC). *Eur. Heart J.* **2023**, *44*, 4043–4140. [CrossRef] [PubMed]
20. Wittwer, J.A.; Golden, S.H.; Joseph, J.J. Diabetes and CVD Risk: Special Considerations in African Americans Related to Care. *Curr. Cardiovasc. Risk Rep.* **2020**, *14*, 15. [CrossRef]
21. Husain, M.; Bain, S.C.; Jeppesen, O.K.; Lingvay, I.; Sørrig, R.; Treppendahl, M.B.; Vilsbøll, T. Semaglutide (SUSTAIN and PIONEER) Reduces Cardiovascular Events in Type 2 Diabetes across Varying Cardiovascular Risk. *Diabetes Obes. Metab.* **2020**, *22*, 442–451. [CrossRef] [PubMed]
22. Ahrén, B.; Masmiquel, L.; Kumar, H.; Sargin, M.; Karsbøl, J.D.; Jacobsen, S.H.; Chow, F. Efficacy and Safety of Once-Weekly Semaglutide versus Once-Daily Sitagliptin as an Add-on to Metformin, Thiazolidinediones, or Both, in Patients with Type 2 Diabetes (SUSTAIN 2): A 56-Week, Double-Blind, Phase 3a, Randomised Trial. *Lancet Diabetes Endocrinol.* **2017**, *5*, 341–354. [CrossRef] [PubMed]
23. Ahmann, A.J.; Capehorn, M.; Charpentier, G.; Dotta, F.; Henkel, E.; Lingvay, I.; Holst, A.G.; Annett, M.P.; Aroda, V.R. Efficacy and Safety of Once-Weekly Semaglutide Versus Exenatide ER in Subjects with Type 2 Diabetes (SUSTAIN 3): A 56-Week, Open-Label, Randomized Clinical Trial. *Diabetes Care* **2017**, *41*, 258–266. [CrossRef]
24. Aroda, V.R.; Bain, S.C.; Cariou, B.; Piletič, M.; Rose, L.; Axelsen, M.; Rowe, E.; DeVries, J.H. Efficacy and Safety of Once-Weekly Semaglutide versus Once-Daily Insulin Glargine as Add-on to Metformin (with or without Sulfonylureas) in Insulin-Naive Patients with Type 2 Diabetes (SUSTAIN 4): A Randomised, Open-Label, Parallel-Group, Multicentre, Multinational, Phase 3a Trial. *Lancet Diabetes Endocrinol.* **2017**, *5*, 355–366. [CrossRef]
25. Sorli, C.; Harashima, S.-I.; Tsoukas, G.M.; Unger, J.; Karsbøl, J.D.; Hansen, T.; Bain, S.C. Efficacy and Safety of Once-Weekly Semaglutide Monotherapy versus Placebo in Patients with Type 2 Diabetes (SUSTAIN 1): A Double-Blind, Randomised, Placebo-Controlled, Parallel-Group, Multinational, Multicentre Phase 3a Trial. *Lancet Diabetes Endocrinol.* **2017**, *5*, 251–260. [CrossRef] [PubMed]
26. Rodbard, H.W.; Lingvay, I.; Reed, J.; de la Rosa, R.; Rose, L.; Sugimoto, D.; Araki, E.; Chu, P.-L.; Wijayasinghe, N.; Norwood, P. Semaglutide Added to Basal Insulin in Type 2 Diabetes (SUSTAIN 5): A Randomized, Controlled Trial. *J. Clin. Endocrinol. Metab.* **2018**, *103*, 2291–2301. [CrossRef] [PubMed]
27. Dziopa, K.; Asselbergs, F.W.; Gratton, J.; Chaturvedi, N.; Schmidt, A.F. Cardiovascular Risk Prediction in Type 2 Diabetes: A Comparison of 22 Risk Scores in Primary Care Settings. *Diabetologia* **2022**, *65*, 644–656. [CrossRef] [PubMed]
28. Damaskos, C.; Garmpis, N.; Kollia, P.; Mitsiopoulos, G.; Barlampa, D.; Drosos, A.; Patsouras, A.; Gravvanis, N.; Antoniou, V.; Litos, A.; et al. Assessing Cardiovascular Risk in Patients with Diabetes: An Update. *Curr. Cardiol. Rev.* **2021**, *16*, 266–274. [CrossRef] [PubMed]
29. Zhang, H.; Qin, L.; Sheng, C.-S.; Niu, Y.; Gu, H.; Lu, S.; Yang, Z.; Tian, J.; Su, Q. ASCVD Risk Stratification Modifies the Effect of HbA1c on Cardiovascular Events among Patients with Type 2 Diabetes Mellitus with Basic to Moderate Risk. *BMJ Open Diabetes Res. Care* **2020**, *8*, e000810. [CrossRef] [PubMed]
30. Vuksan-Ćusa, B.; Jakšić, N.; Matovinović, M.; Baretić, M.; Vuksan-Ćusa, Z.; Mustač, F.; Tudor, K.I.; Šagud, M.; Marčinko, D. Depression and Hopelessness as Possible Predictors of Weight-Change among Obese Day-Hospital Patients: A 6-Months Follow-Up Study. *Psychiatr. Danub.* **2020**, *32*, 217–218. [PubMed]
31. Lim, S.L.; Ong, K.W.; Johal, J.; Han, C.Y.; Yap, Q.V.; Chan, Y.H.; Chooi, Y.C.; Zhang, Z.P.; Chandra, C.C.; Thiagarajah, A.G.; et al. Effect of a Smartphone App on Weight Change and Metabolic Outcomes in Asian Adults with Type 2 Diabetes: A Randomized Clinical Trial. *JAMA Netw. Open* **2021**, *4*, e2112417. [CrossRef] [PubMed]
32. Mustač, F.; Tomašić, L.; Peček, M.; Galijašević, T.; Grkinić, A.; Medić, F.; Matovinović, M.; Marčinko, D. Mobile Applications and Improving the Quality of Life in People with Obesity. In Proceedings of the 2022 7th International Conference on Smart and Sustainable Technologies (SpliTech), Split/Bol, Croatia, 5–8 July 2022; pp. 1–5.
33. Castelnuovo, G.; Pietrabissa, G.; Manzoni, G.M.; Cattivelli, R.; Rossi, A.; Novelli, M.; Varallo, G.; Molinari, E. Cognitive behavioral therapy to aid weight loss in obese patients: Current perspectives. *Psychol. Res. Behav. Manag.* **2017**, *10*, 165–173. [CrossRef]
34. Akhaury, K.; Chaware, S. Relation between Diabetes and Psychiatric Disorders. *Cureus* **2022**, *14*, e30733. [CrossRef]
35. Krejčí, H.; Vyjídák, J.; Kohutiar, M. Low-Carbohydrate Diet in Diabetes Mellitus Treatment. *Vnitr. Lek.* **2018**, *64*, 742–752. [CrossRef]
36. Magkos, F.; Mittendorfer, B. Editorial: Type 2 Diabetes Therapeutics: Weight Loss and Other Strategies. *Curr. Opin. Clin. Nutr. Metab. Care* **2022**, *25*, 256–259. [CrossRef]
37. Sandouk, Z.; Lansang, M.C. Diabetes with Obesity—Is There an Ideal Diet? *Cleve. Clin. J. Med.* **2017**, *84*, S4–S14. [CrossRef]
38. Zang, B.-Y.; He, L.-X.; Xue, L. Intermittent Fasting: Potential Bridge of Obesity and Diabetes to Health? *Nutrients* **2022**, *14*, 981. [CrossRef]

Disclaimer/Publisher's Note: The statements, opinions and data contained in all publications are solely those of the individual author(s) and contributor(s) and not of MDPI and/or the editor(s). MDPI and/or the editor(s) disclaim responsibility for any injury to people or property resulting from any ideas, methods, instructions or products referred to in the content.

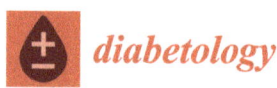 diabetology

Article

Comorbidity of Type 2 Diabetes and Dementia among Hospitalized Patients in Los Angeles County: Hospitalization Outcomes and Costs, 2019–2021

D'Artagnan M. Robinson [1,2], Dalia Regos-Stewart [2], Mariana A. Reyes [2], Tony Kuo [3,4,5] and Noel C. Barragan [2,*]

1. Department of Epidemiology and Biostatistics, Susan and Henry Samueli College of Health Sciences, University of California, Irvine, CA 92617, USA; drobinson2@ph.lacounty.gov
2. Division of Chronic Disease and Injury Prevention, Los Angeles County Department of Public Health, Los Angeles, CA 90010, USA; dregosstewart@ph.lacounty.gov (D.R.-S.); mreyes@ph.lacounty.gov (M.A.R.)
3. Department of Family Medicine, David Geffen School of Medicine, University of California, Los Angeles (UCLA), Los Angeles, CA 90024, USA; tkuo@mednet.ucla.edu
4. Department of Epidemiology, Fielding School of Public Health, University of California, Los Angeles (UCLA), Los Angeles, CA 90095, USA
5. Population Health Program, Clinical and Translational Science Institute, University of California, Los Angeles (UCLA), Los Angeles, CA 90095, USA
* Correspondence: nbarragan@ph.lacounty.gov

Citation: Robinson, D.M.; Regos-Stewart, D.; Reyes, M.A.; Kuo, T.; Barragan, N.C. Comorbidity of Type 2 Diabetes and Dementia among Hospitalized Patients in Los Angeles County: Hospitalization Outcomes and Costs, 2019–2021. *Diabetology* 2023, 4, 586–599. https://doi.org/10.3390/diabetology4040052

Academic Editor: Bernd Stratmann

Received: 11 October 2023
Revised: 23 November 2023
Accepted: 14 December 2023
Published: 18 December 2023

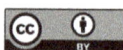

Copyright: © 2023 by the authors. Licensee MDPI, Basel, Switzerland. This article is an open access article distributed under the terms and conditions of the Creative Commons Attribution (CC BY) license (https://creativecommons.org/licenses/by/4.0/).

Abstract: Hospitalizations for diabetes and dementia can impose a significant health and economic toll on older adults in the United States. This study sought to examine differences in hospitalization characteristics and outcomes associated with diabetes and dementia, separately and together, using 2019–2021 discharge record data from the California Department of Health Care Access and Information. The sampled group were residents of Los Angeles County who were aged 50+ at the time of the study. The multivariable linear regression analysis showed that compared to those with no diabetes or dementia, patients with diabetes alone exhibited the highest total charges, while those with comorbid diabetes and dementia exhibited lower charges ($p < 0.05$). The multinomial logistic regression found that patients with comorbid diabetes and dementia had the highest odds of having a length of stay of 7+ days (Adjusted Odds Ratio = 1.49; 95% Confidence Interval (CI) = 1.44–1.53). A matched case–control analysis revealed that comorbid diabetes and dementia were associated with significantly lower odds of hypertensive disease than diabetes alone (Matched Odds Ratio = 0.81; 95% CI = 0.67–0.97). Collectively, these results highlight the complex factors that may influence the variable hospitalization outcomes that are common occurrences in these three distinct disease profiles. Study findings suggest a need to consider these complexities when developing policies or strategies to improve hospitalization outcomes for these conditions.

Keywords: diabetes; Alzheimer's disease; dementia; hospitalization

1. Introduction

Approximately 37 million Americans (11.3% of the United States [US] population) have diabetes [1]. The disease is the eighth leading cause of death nationwide and in 2021 alone was responsible for 103,294 deaths [2]. The vast majority (90–95%) of Americans with diabetes have type 2 diabetes, a condition that inhibits the body from processing blood sugar due to insulin resistance [3]. Type 2 diabetes (hereafter referred to as 'diabetes') most often develops in people over the age of 45; its prevalence increases with age [3,4].

In the US, more than 25% of adults over the age of 65 have diabetes [5]. This higher prevalence in this population has been attributed to age-related changes in organ function and body composition. Among older adults, diabetes has historically been associated with an increased risk of vascular complications, including coronary heart disease, stroke, diabetic kidney disease, retinopathy, and peripheral neuropathy [6]. In recent years, research has identified emerging complications affecting older adults with diabetes, such as various cancers, infections, and diseases of the liver, and dementia and cognitive impairment [6].

Dementia is an umbrella term for changes in cognition due to physiological conditions such as Alzheimer's disease, vascular dementia, and various other illnesses affecting the brain [6]. Numerous studies have found that individuals with diabetes are at an increased risk for developing dementia [6,7]. Furthermore, they have also shown that diabetics with mild cognitive impairment have an increased risk of progressing to dementia [6]. Clinical pathways that may contribute to this relationship include impaired insulin signaling, inflammation, and hypoglycemia [7].

Research has dedicated considerable attention to the burden and cost of diabetes-related hospital care with a focus on potentially avoidable hospitalizations (PAHs) for ambulatory-care-sensitive conditions. Diabetes hospitalization costs have been increasing over the past two decades, which has been attributed, in part, to PAHs for uncontrolled diabetes, short- and long-term diabetic complications, and lower extremity amputations [8]. From 2001 to 2014, the national cost of PAHs related to diabetes increased from USD 4.5 billion to USD 5.9 billion. The majority (75%) of this increase was due to a rise in diabetes-related PAHs, with the remainder being attributed to an increase in mean cost per admission.

Hospitalizations also played a significant role in driving the healthcare costs of dementia over the years [9,10]. Lin and colleagues found that in 2013 alone, the total cost of hospitalizations for Medicare beneficiaries with dementia was USD 4.7 billion [10]. They also found that nearly one in ten of these patients were hospitalized for a potentially avoidable condition, and that nearly one in five had an unplanned readmission within 30 days. A state-wide matched analysis of Medicare costs in Tennessee by Husaini and colleagues found that hospitalization costs were 14% higher among dementia patients as compared to patients without dementia; those with dementia also had a significantly higher frequency of diabetes (36% vs. 32%, $p < 0.001$) [9].

Individuals with both diabetes and dementia are known to be at an increased risk for PAHs. A 2017 study by Lin et al., which examined Medicare claims data, found that patients with dementia were more likely to have PAHs for short- and long-term diabetic complications than patients without dementia [11]. Another study by Zaslavsky et al. found that incident dementia was associated with increased rates of hospitalization among individuals with diabetes, both for diabetic complications and non-diabetic complications, such as dehydration or urinary tract infections [12]. While there is a growing body of research focused on the risk for and outcomes of PAHs among individuals with comorbid diabetes and dementia, few studies have provided in-depth comparisons of the demographic and health characteristics of patients with diabetes, with dementia, and with diabetes and dementia together. To the best of our knowledge, no studies have examined the differences in cost and duration of hospitalization and costs for individuals with these three distinct health profiles.

To address this gap in the literature, we analyzed Los Angeles County hospital discharge data from 2019 to 2021 to better understand the factors affecting hospitalizations of individuals with diabetes, with dementia, and with both conditions together (comorbidity). This study sought to (1) describe the differences in demographic and hospitalization characteristics and outcomes, including costs, between these groups; (2) examine the factors that may influence total charges and hospital length of stay; and (3) compare the odds of diabetic complications for individuals with comorbid diabetes and dementia versus those with only diabetes.

2. Materials and Methods

2.1. Data Source and Study Population

Hospitalizations were examined using patient discharge data (PDD) for the years 2019–2021 derived from the California Department of Health Care Access and Information (HCAI) [13]. HCAI maintains non-public, limited data sets consisting of patient-level inpatient discharge data collected from all state-licensed hospitals in California. Licensed hospitals include general acute care, acute psychiatric, chemical dependency recovery, and psychiatric health facilities. PDD contains demographic, clinical, payer, and facility data for all inpatient records. HCAI datasets do not contain any direct identifiers (i.e., name, address, social security number); additional safeguards are typically implemented to ensure that dataset information could not be used to personally identify individuals (e.g., avoiding cell counts smaller than 12).

All hospitalizations of Los Angeles County residents aged 50 years and older at the time of admission were included in the present analysis (n = 1,472,688), reflecting 47% of all hospitalization records during the study period (n = 3,160,404). The analysis sample was stratified into four mutually exclusive groups based on disease status: (i) diabetes, (ii) dementia, (iii) diabetes and dementia, and (iv) no diabetes or dementia. Disease status was classified using the International Classification of Diseases, Tenth Revision, Clinical Modifications (ICD-10-CM) codes (see Supplemental Table S1) [14]. Diagnosis of diabetes and/or dementia was established based on the listing of a diabetes or dementia ICD-10-CM code as (a) the chief cause of admission of the patient for hospital care or (b) a coexisting condition at the time of admission that developed during the hospital stay, or that affected the treatment received and/or the length of stay of the hospitalization. Individuals with dementia were defined as having one of the following relevant diagnoses: Alzheimer's disease, vascular dementia, dementia in other diseases classified elsewhere, unspecified dementia, Huntington's disease, Parkinson's disease, other secondary Parkinsonism, frontotemporal dementia, Pick's disease, other frontotemporal neurocognitive disorder, senile degeneration of the brain not elsewhere classified, and/or neurocognitive disorder with Lewy bodies.

2.2. Variables

To understand the characteristics of hospitalizations by disease status, descriptive and univariate statistics were generated for the following variables: length of stay—the total number of days from admission to discharge date; total charges—the total charges for services rendered based on the hospital's full established rates, in US dollars; age; sex; race/ethnicity; year of hospital admission; disposition—the consequent arrangement or event ending the patient's stay in the hospital; type of care—the licensure of the bed occupied by the patient; expected source of payment—the entity or organization expected to pay the greatest share of the patient's bill such as Medicare or private coverage; type of admission, such as emergency or elective; and source of admission—site where the patient originated such as a non-healthcare facility of different hospital facility.

Length of stay, total charges, and age were examined as continuous variables. Race/ethnicity was categorized as White, Black, Hispanic, Asian, and Other (inclusive of Other, American Indian/Alaskan Native, Native Hawaiian or Other Pacific Islander, and Multiracial). Disposition was categorized in alignment with categories established in the Agency for Healthcare Research and Quality's Healthcare Cost & Utilization Project as routine discharge, transfer to a short-term hospital, transfer to other (inclusive of skilled nursing facilities (SNF), intermediate care facilities (ICF), and other types of facilities), home healthcare, against medical advice, and died [15]. The type of care was categorized as acute care or other types of care (inclusive of skilled nursing care/intermediate care, psychiatric care, chemical dependency recovery care, and physical rehabilitation care) for this analysis. The expected source of payment was categorized as Medicare, Medi-Cal (California's Medicaid program), private coverage, and other (inclusive of workers' compensation, county indigent programs, other government, other indigent, self-pay, or other). The type of admission was categorized as emergency, urgent, elective, or trauma. Finally, the source of admission was categorized as non-healthcare facility, clinic/physician's office, different hospital facility, SNF/ICF/assisted living facility (ALF), or other (inclusive of court/law enforcement sites, one distinct unit to another distinct unit of the same hospital, ambulatory surgery centers, hospices, and designated disaster alternate care sites). Additionally, because the study period coincided with the onset and peak of the coronavirus disease 2019 (COVID-19) pandemic, which had a significant impact on hospitalizations across the US, diagnosis of COVID-19 was also examined [16–18].

2.3. Total Charges

A multiple linear regression model was constructed for total charges incurred for all services rendered during the patient's hospitalization. To satisfy the normality assumption for linear regression modelling, the dependent variable was log-transformed, and 1 was subsequently added to stabilize the log-transformed variable to account for instances of zero values for total charges. The total charge variable was regressed on disease status, age, sex, race/ethnicity, year of hospital admission, disposition, type of care, expected source of payment, type of admission, source of admission, and COVID-19 diagnosis.

Best subsets, backwards, and stepwise selection algorithms were utilized with the Akaike information criterion (AIC), Bayesian information criterion (BIC), and adjusted R-squared noted for all approaches to determine the best-fitted model; the practical and clinical relevancy of the variables to be included were also considered. In the model building, all three algorithms selected all variables of interest for inclusion in the final model. The model was then checked for potentially influential outliers utilizing statistical measures of influence; based on the results, no observations were deleted. The normality of residuals was also assessed using a histogram overlayed with a kernel density and normal plot. Finally, homoskedasticity was assessed using the studentized residuals vs. fitted values plot. No violations of any model assumptions were detected.

Discharge records with any missing or invalid data for the log total charge variable or any of the covariates were excluded from the analysis. The total sample size included in the final linear model was $n = 1,450,843$. Parameter estimates and 95% confidence intervals (CIs) were generated, and the statistical significance threshold was set at $p < 0.05$.

2.4. Length of Stay

A multinomial logistic regression model was built for length of stay, which was categorized by quartiles: 0–1 days, 2–3 days, 4–6 days, and 7+ days. Despite the ordinal nature of the length of stay variable, it was analyzed as a non-ordered multinomial variable due to a violation of the proportional odds assumption. Length of stay was regressed on disease status, age category (50–59 years, 60–69 years, 70–79 years, 80–89 years, and 90+ years), sex, race/ethnicity, year of hospital admission, disposition, type of care, expected source of payment, type of admission, source of admission, and COVID-19 diagnosis.

Forward and backward selection algorithms were used to test variable selection. The model fit was assessed using objective functions like likelihood ratio test measures, AIC, and BIC; as with the multiple linear regression model, the practical and clinical relevancy of identified variables were also considered. In the model building, both algorithms selected all variables of interest for inclusion in the final model. Model checking included an assessment of multicollinearity by measuring Cramer's V for each pair of categorical variables. The absence of complete separation was ascertained by checking standard errors and parameter estimates for extremely large and/or infinite values. No violations of any multinomial logistic models were detected.

Discharges that had any missing or invalid data for the length of stay variable or any of the covariates were excluded from the analysis. The total sample size included in the final multinomial model was $n = 1,450,843$. Adjusted odds ratios (AORs) and 95% CIs were generated, and the statistical significance threshold was set at $p < 0.05$.

2.5. Matched Case–Control Analysis

To explore the differences in odds of diabetic complications experienced by those with comorbid diabetes and dementia compared to those with diabetes alone, a 1:4 matched, nested case–control analysis was employed. From the pool of discharge records with complete data ($n = 1,450,843$), cases (those with diabetes and dementia) and controls (those with diabetes alone) were selected and matched based on the year of hospital admission, sex, age, and race/ethnicity. The final matched sample size consisted of 1492 cases and 5968 controls.

Univariate and descriptive statistics for cases and controls were examined for length of stay, total charges, age, sex, race/ethnicity, year of hospital admission, dispositions, type of care, expected sources of payment (categorized as Medicare, Medi-Cal, and other), type of admission (categorized as emergency, urgent, and other), and source of admission.

Conditional logistic regression models were employed to assess the likelihood of hospitalization for five diabetic complications for cases compared to controls. Complications examined included the following: ophthalmic complications; kidney complications; neurological complications; hypertensive diseases; and lower-extremity amputations (based on ICD-10-Procedural Coding System classification; see Supplemental Table S1). Matched odds ratios (MORs) and 95% CIs were generated for each model; the statistical significance threshold was set at $p < 0.05$.

After evaluating for potential confounders, no sizable impacts to the crude MOR estimates were detected; therefore, regression models were unadjusted. Model checking included an assessment of the linearity between the log odds of the diabetic complications and age; outlier influence assessment and case-wise deletion procedures; and confirmation of the efficiency of the matching process.

All statistical analyses were conducted using SAS analytical software version 9.4 (SAS Institute Inc., Cary, NC, USA). This study was considered exempt as non-human-subject research by the Los Angeles County Department of Public Health Institutional Review Board.

3. Results

During the 3-year study period, a total of 523,987 discharges (36.7%) were indicated as having diabetes and incurred a total of USD 62.5 billion in total charges; 32,376 of these discharges listed diabetes as the chief cause of admission. A total of 115,958 (8.1%) had dementia and incurred a total of USD 11.8 billion in total charges; of these, approximately 5% ($n = 5849$) listed dementia as the chief cause of admission. Approximately 5.5% of patients had both ($n = 78,088$) diabetes and dementia and incurred a total of USD 8.7 billion in hospital charges. The median length of stay and total charges were highest among those with comorbid diabetes and dementia—5 days and USD 71,398, respectively (Table 1). The median age at admission was found to be highest among patients with dementia alone (84 years). Differences by sex were most pronounced among those with dementia alone, with females being more frequently diagnosed with dementia (55.0%) as compared to males (45.0%). Race/ethnicity patterns varied significantly by disease status. For example, among those with diabetes alone, Hispanics comprised the largest group (43.6%), and among those with comorbid diabetes and dementia, those classified as Other made up the largest group (51.0%). Notably, disposition upon discharge varied substantially, with far fewer patients with dementia (alone or in conjunction with diabetes) having a routine discharge (e.g., 18.2% of those with dementia compared to 48.2% of those with diabetes). Across all disease categories, Medicare was the primary source of payment for the majority of inpatients and most admissions were characterized as emergency admissions originating from non-healthcare facility sources (e.g., patients' homes). The frequency of COVID-19 diagnoses was highest among individuals with comorbid diabetes and dementia (7.1%).

Multivariable linear regression revealed that individuals with diabetes alone exhibited 8.9% [$\exp(\beta_1) - 1 = \exp(-0.115) - 1$] higher total charges when compared to individuals without dementia or diabetes, while holding all other variables constant ($p < 0.0001$); see Table 2. Conversely, those with dementia or comorbid diabetes and dementia had lower total charges (-10.9% and -2.9%, respectively; $p < 0.0001$).

Table 1. Hospital Discharges by Disease Status, Los Angeles County, 2019–2021.

Characteristics	Median [Range] or N (%)				
	Diabetes (n = 523,987)	Dementia (n = 115,958)	Diabetes + Dementia (n = 78,088)	No Diabetes or Dementia (n = 754,655)	p-Value [1]
Length of Stay (days)	4 [0–900]	4 [0–807]	5 [0–938]	3 [0–859]	<0.0001
Total Charges (USD)	$68,378 [$0–$10,795,377]	$65,297 [$0–$7,067,876]	$71,398 [$0–$5,087,514]	$63,641 [$0–$12,281,262]	<0.0001
Age (years)	68 [50–119]	84 [50–116]	82 [50–109]	67 [50–120]	<0.0001
Sex					<0.0001
Male	275,695 (52.6)	49,939 (45.0)	35,125 (49.8)	376,559 (49.9)	
Female	248,272 (47.4)	66,018 (55.0)	42,962 (50.2)	378,056 (50.1)	
Race/Ethnicity					<0.0001
White	134,014 (25.9)	56,118 (31.5)	323,871 (43.3)	321,829 (43.2)	
Black	69,370 (13.4)	13,498 (14.3)	97,841 (13.0)	96,996 (13.0)	
Hispanic	226,117 (43.6)	23,050 (31.5)	210,541 (28.0)	208,257 (28.0)	
Asian	55,107 (10.6)	13,771 (15.4)	70,157 (9.3)	69,715 (9.3)	
Other [2]	33,588 (6.5)	7821 (7.2)	48,595 (51.0)	48,213 (6.5)	
Year of Hospital Admission					<0.0001
2019	183,917 (35.1)	43,014 (37.1)	28,053 (35.9)	278,218 (36.9)	
2020	168,655 (32.2)	37,993 (32.8)	26,355 (33.8)	235,295 (31.2)	
2021	171,415 (32.7)	34,951 (30.1)	23,680 (30.3)	241,142 (31.9)	
Disposition					<0.0001
Routine	252,600 (48.2)	21,034 (18.2)	13,877 (17.8)	403,272 (53.5)	
Transfer to Short-Term Hospital	19,211 (3.7)	3499 (3.0)	2491 (3.2)	23,165 (3.1)	
Transfer Other [3]	95,661 (18.3)	54,486 (47.1)	37,166 (47.6)	119,420 (15.8)	
Home Healthcare	119,312 (22.8)	27,107 (23.4)	17,566 (22.5)	159,367 (21.1)	
Against Medical Advice	10,510 (2.0)	1215 (1.1)	850 (1.1)	17,591 (2.3)	
Died	26,531 (5.1)	8318 (7.2)	6109 (7.8)	31,635 (4.2)	
Type of Care					<0.0001
Acute Care	500,009 (95.4)	107,152 (92.4)	73,698 (94.4)	698,036 (92.5)	
Other [4]	23,947 (0.9)	8795 (1.6)	4383 (1.4)	56,562 (0.9)	
Expected Source of Payment					<0.0001
Medicare	315,441 (60.2)	101,431 (87.5)	67,753 (86.8)	417,368 (55.3)	
Medi-Cal (Medicaid)	121,779 (23.3)	7901 (6.8)	6463 (8.3)	156,409 (20.7)	
Private Coverage	74,479 (14.2)	5710 (4.9)	3361 (4.3)	155,542 (20.6)	
Other [5]	12,067 (2.3)	881 (0.8)	495 (0.6)	24,981 (3.3)	
Type of Admission					<0.0001
Emergency	297,508 (56.8)	69,839 (60.2)	48,423 (62.0)	379,635 (50.3)	
Urgent	154,218 (29.4)	34,610 (29.9)	22,533 (28.9)	212,778 (28.2)	
Elective	69,049 (13.2)	10,493 (9.1)	6672 (8.5)	153,580 (20.4)	
Trauma	3011 (0.6)	979 (0.8)	447 (0.6)	8431 (1.1)	
Source of Admission					<0.0001
Non-Healthcare Facility	418,371 (80.0)	76,149 (65.8)	50,492 (64.8)	602,401 (79.9)	
Clinic/Physician's Office	17,941 (3.4)	1941 (1.7)	1164 (1.5)	32,408 (4.3)	
Hospital (Different Facility)	49,867 (9.5)	12,550 (10.8)	8704 (11.2)	72,284 (9.6)	
SNF/ICF/ALF	22,401 (4.3)	20,561 (17.8)	14,947 (19.2)	24,626 (3.3)	
Other [6]	14,604 (2.8)	4551 (3.9)	2639 (3.4)	21,850 (2.9)	
COVID-19 Diagnosis					<0.0001
Confirmed Diagnosis	36,230 (6.9)	7112 (6.1)	5541 (7.1)	34,408 (4.6)	
No Confirmed Diagnosis	487,757 (93.1)	108,846 (93.9)	72,547 (92.9)	720,247 (95.4)	

Key: ALF = assisted living facility; ICF = intermediate care facility; SNF = skilled nursing facility; USD = United States Dollar. Percentages may not add to 100% due to rounding. Frequency counts for a given variable may not sum to a column total due to missing data or invalid variable codes. [1] p-values generated using Kruskal–Wallis and chi-squared tests. [2] Includes: Other, American Indian/Alaskan Native, Native Hawaiian or Other Pacific Islander, and Multiracial. [3] Includes: SNF, ICF, other types of facilities. [4] Includes: skilled nursing care/intermediate care, psychiatric care, chemical dependency recovery care, and physical rehabilitation care. [5] Includes: workers' compensation, county indigent programs, other government, other indigent, self-pay, and other. [6] Includes: court/law enforcement sites, one distinct unit to another distinct unit of the same hospital, ambulatory surgery centers, hospices, and designated disaster alternate care sites.

Table 2. Multivariable Linear Regression Analysis—Log Total Charges Billed for Hospitalizations by Disease Status, Los Angeles County, 2019–2021.

Covariate	Parameter Estimate	95% Confidence Interval	p-Value
Disease Status (Referent: No Diabetes or Dementia)			
Diabetes	0.085	(0.082, 0.089)	<0.0001
Dementia	−0.115	(−0.121, −0.109)	<0.0001
Diabetes + Dementia	−0.029	(−0.036, −0.022)	<0.0001

Multinomial logistic regression examining length of stay revealed that relative to those who were hospitalized for 0–1 days, patients with comorbid diabetes and dementia had the highest odds of a 2–3 day length of stay (AOR = 1.20, 95% CI = 1.17–1.24), with other predictor variables in the model held constant; see Table 3. Model estimates for a length of stay of 4–6 days and 7+ days revealed parallel patterns.

Table 3. Multinomial Logistic Regression Analysis—Length of Stay and of Hospital Discharges by Disease Status on Length of Stay, Los Angeles County, 2019–2021.

Length of Stay in Days Categorized by Quartiles (Referent Group: 0–1 Days)			
Length of Stay Groups	2–3 Days	4–6 Days	7+ Days
	Adjusted OR (95% CI)	Adjusted OR (95% CI)	Adjusted OR (95% CI)
Disease Status (Referent: No Diabetes or Dementia)			
Diabetes	1.12 (1.11–1.13) *	1.22 (1.21–1.24) *	1.33 (1.31–1.34) *
Dementia	1.15 (1.13–1.18) *	1.25 (1.22–1.28) *	1.22 (1.20–1.26) *
Diabetes + Dementia	1.20 (1.17–1.24) *	1.42 (1.38–1.46) *	1.49 (1.44–1.53) *

* $p < 0.05$.

After matching, patients with comorbid diabetes and dementia exhibited significant differences across all variables of interest, with the exception of total charges (Table 4).

Table 4. Hospital Discharge Characteristics of Matched Cases (diabetes and dementia) and Controls (diabetes alone), Los Angeles County, 2019–2021.

Characteristics	Median [Range] or N (%)		
	Cases (n = 1492)	Controls (n = 5968)	p-Value [1]
Length of Stay (days)	5 [0–366]	4 [0–122]	<0.0001
Total Charges (USD)	$77,772 [$4665–$2,657,694]	$74,818 [$0–$2,011,253]	0.38
Age (years)	75.5 [50–103]	75.5 [50–103]	1.0
Sex			1.0
Male	737 (45.0)	2948 (52.7)	
Female	755 (55.0)	3020 (47.3)	
Race/Ethnicity			1.0
White	315 (31.1)	1260 (25.5)	
Black	300 (14.1)	1200 (13.2)	
Hispanic	309 (31.0)	1236 (43.2)	
Asian	289 (15.2)	1156 (10.6)	
Other [2]	279 (0.1)	1116 (0.2)	

Table 4. *Cont.*

Characteristics	Median [Range] or N (%)		p-Value [1]
	Cases (n = 1492)	Controls (n = 5968)	
Year of Hospital Admission			1.0
2019	499 (35.9)	1996 (35.0)	
2020	494 (33.8)	1976 (32.2)	
2021	499 (30.3)	1996 (32.7)	
Disposition			<0.0001
Routine	284 (19.0)	2642 (44.3)	
Transfer to Short-Term Hospital	40 (2.7)	221 (3.7)	
Transfer Other [3]	782 (52.4)	1307 (21.9)	
Home Healthcare	246 (16.5)	1268 (21.2)	
Against Medical Advice	12 (0.8)	132 (2.2)	
Died	128 (8.6)	398 (6.7)	
Type of Care			<0.0001
Acute Care	1409 (94.4)	5706 (95.6)	
Other [4]	83 (5.6)	262 (4.4)	
Expected Source of Payment			<0.0001
Medicare	1128 (75.6)	3884 (65.1)	
Medi-Cal	220 (14.7)	1083 (18.2)	
Other [5]	143 (9.6)	997 (16.7)	
Type of Admission			<0.0001
Emergency	908 (60.9)	3223 (54.0)	
Urgent	467 (31.3)	2114 (35.4)	
Other [6]	117 (7.8)	630 (10.6)	
Source of Admission			<0.0001
Non-Healthcare Facility	895 (60.0)	4823 (80.8)	
Clinic/Physician's Office	22 (1.5)	170 (2.8)	
Hospital (Different Facility)	187 (12.5)	528 (8.8)	
SNF/ICF/ALF	357 (23.9)	296 (4.9)	
Other [7]	31 (2.1)	151 (3.0)	
COVID-19 Diagnosis			0.15
Confirmed Diagnosis	105 (7.0)	360 (6.0)	
No Confirmed Diagnosis	1387 (93.0)	5608 (94.0)	

Key: ALF = assisted living facility; ICF = intermediate care facility; SNF = skilled nursing facility; USD = United States Dollar. Percentages may add to less or more than 100% due to rounding. [1] p-values generated using Kruskal–Wallis and chi-squared tests. [2] Includes: Other, American Indian/Alaskan Native, Native Hawaiian or Other Pacific Islander, and Multiracial. [3] Includes: SNF, ICF, and other types of facilities. [4] Includes: skilled nursing care/intermediate care, psychiatric care, chemical dependency recovery care, and physical rehabilitation care. [5] Includes: workers' compensation, county indigent programs, other government, other indigent, self-pay, and other. [6] Includes: elective and trauma. [7] Includes: court/law enforcement sites, one distinct unit to another distinct unit of the same hospital, ambulatory surgery centers, hospices, and designated disaster alternate care sites.

Conditional logistic regression analyses revealed that there were minimal differences in diabetic complications among those with comorbid diabetes and dementia as compared to those with dementia, with the exception of hypertensive diseases (Table 5). Comorbid diabetes and dementia were associated with a decreased risk of hypertensive diseases (OR = 0.81, 95% CI = 0.67–0.97).

Table 5. Crude Conditional Logistic Regression Analyses—Associations Between Disease Status and Diabetic Complications Among Hospitalizations in Los Angeles County, 2019–2021.

Diabetic Complications	Matched Odds Ratio	95% Confidence Interval	p-Value
Kidney Complications	1.04	0.92–1.18	0.49
Ophthalmic Complications	0.69	0.47–1.02	0.06
Neurologic Complications	1.00	0.80–1.27	0.98
Hypertensive Diseases	0.81	0.67–0.97	0.02
Low-Extremity Amputation Procedures	1.36	0.73–2.55	0.33

4. Discussion

Previous studies have explored the economic burden of and factors influencing hospitalizations among patients with diabetes, dementia, and their associated comorbidities [8,9,19,20]. However, these studies have primarily focused on a single disease profile, such as diabetes or dementia, or examined the two as part of a more general description of comorbidities. Our study specifically sought to build upon this research by providing a more comprehensive understanding of the health profiles of hospitalized patients in Los Angeles County who had comorbid diabetes and dementia. Four takeaways can be gleaned from examining these hospitalization data.

First, patients with comorbid diabetes and dementia experienced longer hospital stays compared to the other groups. This is in keeping with previous research which showed that patients with dementia may require more time to assess and manage comorbidities before discharge, have longer recovery periods more generally, or have increased disease severity, and are often moved to skilled nursing facilities and other post-hospitalization venues for further management [19]. Interestingly, despite patients with diabetes generally having a shorter length of stay, they had the highest total charges, after adjusting for covariates and comparing them to other disease groups. This may be attributed, in part, to high-cost care procedures being implemented in the first days of admission. For example, a study by Fine et al. found that the cost of care for hospitalized patients with pneumonia was lowest on the day of discharge and the 2 days preceding discharge [21]. Furthermore, caregivers of patients with comorbid diabetes and dementia may need further support in learning how to manage their condition, which may extend the length of stay with minimal relative added costs [22]. Increasing age may have also played a role in extending the length of stay in the hospital. In the literature, advanced age has been found to be associated with increases in longer duration of hospitalization; it also correlates with disease severity [23].

Second, our study showed that there were differences in racial and ethnic disparities across the different disease profiles in the HCAI data. This may suggest that health inequities are present in how hospitals detect and manage patients with comorbid diabetes and dementia. Prior research indicates that documentation of a dementia diagnosis is likely distorted in hospitalization records, as dementia diagnoses were often missed or delayed among non-White racial and ethnic groups [24]. For example, non-Hispanic Black adults and Hispanics have been shown to be 27% and 84% more likely, respectively, to have a missed or delayed diagnosis of dementia compared to non-Hispanic whites [24].

These racial and ethnic differences may also be explained by payer category. For instance, prior research has highlighted both lower dementia diagnosis prevalence and incidence rates among Medicare Advantage (MA) beneficiaries versus beneficiaries of traditional Medicare (TM) [25]. MA plans are private options that incentivize the use of preventive services. In 2022, large percentages of racial and ethnic minorities were enrolled in these plans. However, despite MA beneficiaries being more likely to receive annual wellness visits and structured cognitive assessments, as compared to TM beneficiaries, the prevalence of diagnosed dementia (MA = 7.10% vs. TM = 8.70%) and incidence rate for this condition (MA = 2.50% vs. TM = 2.99%) were still lower for these MA beneficiaries [25].

Third, patients with dementia and those with comorbid diabetes and dementia were more frequently transferred to specialized long-term care facilities (e.g., SNF), whereas patients with diabetes alone had more routine discharges. This finding aligns with existing literature showing that transitions to a skilled nursing facility are especially common among patients with dementia [26]. Patients with dementia are more likely to have multiple coexisting chronic conditions, often requiring more complex and intensive care [27]. It could also be the case that the community resources that are geared toward diabetes care are generally more organized and reimbursable than dementia care—this is an area of need where better health policies and interventions should be implemented [28–30].

Fourth, results from the matched case–control analysis suggest that the presence of hypertensive complications was lower among patients with comorbid diabetes and dementia than among patients with diabetes alone. While somewhat counterintuitive since hypertension is a risk factor for dementia, this finding, nonetheless, aligns with other studies that have found an inverse association between dementia and late-life hypertension [31,32]. However, these differences should be interpreted cautiously and within the context of the data source that was used to ascertain the diagnoses—i.e., hospitalization records versus full medical history records. Data derived from hospitalization records may not reflect all diagnoses that relate to earlier hospitalizations or pre-existing medical conditions and they typically do not include information about medication or prescribed treatments. These aspects of the data source may have lowered observations of hypertensive disease in those with both conditions, even though hypertension is an established risk factor for dementia and is known to affect cognition [33–37]. As an example, a systematic review of observational studies found that 73% of those with dementia were taking at least one antihypertensive medication [35].

While our study focuses on the hospital setting specifically, it is essential to recognize that there is a broader healthcare context to this work. For example, emerging evidence suggests that cardiovascular and cerebrovascular disease caused by diabetes are closely associated with the onset of cognitive decline for individuals with these types of vascular etiology [38]. Additionally, the cerebral insulin resistance caused by diabetes has been found to be associated with increased beta-amyloid production and tau protein phosphorylation, two hallmark characteristics of Alzheimer's disease [38]. These potential causal connections highlight the importance of implementing comprehensive healthcare strategies that can take care of both the acute and long-term care needs of patients who have comorbid diabetes and dementia. The complex interplay between these two conditions highlights the need for tailored healthcare policies that can meaningfully address the unique challenges presented by both of these conditions, not only during hospitalization but also in post-acute care settings.

As previously noted, this study coincides with the COVID-19 pandemic, which had a significant impact on hospitalizations, especially for older adults [39]. Age was and is still considered to be the most important risk factor for severe COVID-19 symptoms, with the risk of severe outcomes increasing with advancing age [40]. Diabetes has also been identified as a significant risk factor for severe COVID-19 and subsequent hospitalization [41,42]. A national analysis found that the rate of in-hospital mortality due to COVID-19 was greater among diabetic patients than among non-diabetic patients (16.3% versus 8.1%, $p < 0.0001$) [43]. Emerging literature also suggests that those with dementia are at increased risk for more severe COVID-19 complications, including hospitalization [44,45]. A multivariable logistic regression analysis found increased odds of in-hospital mortality among patients with diabetes and all-cause dementia when they were hospitalized for COVID-19 [46]. Cardiovascular disease and related conditions represent another factor that may have impacted those with diabetes and dementia, as these conditions were found to be associated with greater COVID-19 mortality and intensive care unit admission [47–51].

Limitations

While this study has a number of strengths, including its large sample size and low rate of missing data, it has several limitations. First, discharge records represent unique hospitalizations rather than individuals and do not allow for examination of readmissions after discharge or recurrent hospitalizations. Second, recorded diagnoses related to a prior episode that have no bearing on the current hospital stay were excluded. This may have resulted in an underestimation of patients with diabetes and dementia. Third, the use of ICD-10-CM codes alone to determine the presence of diabetes and dementia. Third, the use of ICD-10-CM codes alone to determine the presence of dementia likely contributed to an underestimation of dementia. Research has shown that many of those who meet the diagnostic criteria for dementia are not diagnosed by a physician [52]. Fourth, the reliance on ICD-10-CM codes to ascertain dementia diagnoses could have led to misclassification bias; as such, incorrect diagnoses may have affected observed estimates. Finally, detailed information on patient risk factors, medical history, and socioeconomic status, which can increase the severity of disease and, correspondingly, hospitalization outcomes, were not available. Without such information, we were unable to adequately adjust for these confounding factors in our analyses.

5. Conclusions

Study findings highlight the substantial healthcare burden associated with comorbid diabetes and dementia. This burden is expected to grow as the number of Americans with these conditions is projected to increase substantially over the next few decades [52–55]. Our results underscore the need for a multi-faceted approach to address both diabetes and dementia, in many instances, concurrently, especially for high-risk populations that lack adequate access to health services, are vulnerable to socioeconomic challenges, and have historically experienced health inequities and barriers to care, including systemic racism [56,57]. Investments in strategies such as preventative care, care coordination, advance care planning, personalized care plans, and community support for improving self-management and caregiver assistance will be critical for mitigating the financial and social impacts of these prevailing and costly chronic diseases [58–64]. These are all areas of health policy research, strategy intervention, and program implementation that will be required to address the comorbidity of diabetes and dementia in Los Angeles County and elsewhere across the US [65–67].

Supplementary Materials: The following supporting information can be downloaded at: https://www.mdpi.com/article/10.3390/diabetology4040052/s1, Table S1: ICD-10-CM and ICD-10-PCS Codes Used.

Author Contributions: Conceptualization, D.M.R., N.C.B. and T.K.; Formal Analysis, D.M.R. and N.CB.; Writing—Original Draft Preparation, D.M.R., D.R.-S. and M.A.R.; Writing—Review and Editing, D.M.R., D.R.-S., M.A.R., T.K. and N.C.B.; Fund Acquisition—N.C.B. All authors have read and agreed to the published version of the manuscript.

Funding: This work was supported in part by funding from the Alzheimer's Association through a cooperative agreement with the Centers for Disease Control and Prevention [NU58DP006744].

Institutional Review Board Statement: This analysis was considered exempt as non-human-subject research per 45 CFR 46.102(e) by the Los Angeles County Department of Public Health Institutional Review Board, Project No. 2023-05-014.

Informed Consent Statement: This project was a secondary data analysis of an existing, deidentified database.

Data Availability Statement: Restrictions apply to the availability of these data. Data were obtained from the California Department of Health Care Access and Information and are available at https://hcai.ca.gov/data-and-reports/request-data/ (accessed on 20 March 2023) to eligible hospitals and health departments with the permission of the California Department of Health Care Access and Information.

Acknowledgments: The findings and conclusions presented in this article are those of the authors and do not necessarily represent the views of the funder, grantee, or any of the other organizations referenced in the text. The authors would like to thank the California Department of Health Care Access and Information for providing access to patient discharge data.

Conflicts of Interest: The authors declare no conflict of interest.

References

1. American Diabetes Association. Statistics about Diabetes. Available online: https://diabetes.org/about-us/statistics/about-diabetes (accessed on 27 September 2023).
2. Centers for Disease Control and Prevention. National Center for Health Statistics. Diabetes. Available online: https://www.cdc.gov/nchs/fastats/diabetes.htm (accessed on 27 September 2023).
3. Centers for Disease Control and Prevention. Type 2 Diabetes. Available online: https://www.cdc.gov/diabetes/basics/type2.html (accessed on 27 September 2023).
4. Saeedi, P.; Petersohn, I.; Salpea, P.; Malanda, B.; Karuranga, S.; Unwin, N.; Colagiuri, S.; Guariguata, L.; Motala, A.; Ogurtsova, K.; et al. Global and Regional Diabetes Prevalence Estimates for 2019 and Projections for 2030 and 2045: Results from the International Diabetes Federation Diabetes Atlas, 9th edition. *Diabetes Res. Clin. Pract.* **2019**, *157*, 107843. [CrossRef] [PubMed]
5. Sesti, G.; Antonelli Incalzi, R.; Bonora, E.; Consoli, A.; Giaccari, A.; Maggi, S.; Paolisso, G.; Purrello, F.; Vendemiale, G.; Ferrara, N. Management of Diabetes in Older Adults. *Nutr. Metab. Cardiovasc. Dis.* **2018**, *28*, 206–218. [CrossRef] [PubMed]
6. Tomic, D.; Shaw, J.E.; Magliano, D.J. The Burden and Risks of Emerging Complications of Diabetes Mellitus. *Nat. Rev. Endocrinol.* **2022**, *18*, 525–539. [CrossRef] [PubMed]
7. Simó, R.; Ciudin, A.; Simó-Servat, O.; Hernández, C. Cognitive Impairment and Dementia: A New Emerging Complication of Type 2 Diabetes-The Diabetologist's Perspective. *Acta Diabetol.* **2017**, *54*, 417–424. [CrossRef] [PubMed]
8. Shrestha, S.S.; Zhang, P.; Hora, I.; Geiss, L.S.; Luman, E.T.; Gregg, E.W. Factors Contributing to Increases in Diabetes-Related Preventable Hospitalization Costs among U.S. Adults During 2001–2014. *Diabetes Care* **2019**, *42*, 77–84. [CrossRef] [PubMed]
9. Husaini, B.; Gudlavalleti, A.S.; Cain, V.; Levine, R.; Moonis, M. Risk Factors and Hospitalization Costs of Dementia Patients: Examining Race and Gender Variations. *Indian J. Community Med.* **2015**, *40*, 258–263. [CrossRef] [PubMed]
10. Lin, P.J.; Zhong, Y.; Fillit, H.M.; Cohen, J.T.; Neumann, P.J. Hospitalizations for Ambulatory Care Sensitive Conditions and Unplanned Readmissions among Medicare Beneficiaries with Alzheimer's Disease. *Alzheimers Dement.* **2017**, *13*, 1174–1178. [CrossRef] [PubMed]
11. Lin, P.J.; Fillit, H.M.; Cohen, J.T.; Neumann, P.J. Potentially Avoidable Hospitalizations among Medicare Beneficiaries with Alzheimer's Disease and Related Disorders. *Alzheimers Dement.* **2013**, *9*, 30–38. [CrossRef]
12. Zaslavsky, O.; Yu, O.; Walker, R.L.; Crane, P.K.; Gray, S.L.; Sadak, T.; Borson, S.; Larson, E.B. Incident Dementia, Glycated Hemoglobin (HbA1c) Levels, and Potentially Preventable Hospitalizations in People Aged 65 and Older with Diabetes. *J. Gerontol. A Biol. Sci. Med. Sci.* **2021**, *76*, 2054–2061. [CrossRef]
13. California Department of Health Care Access and Information. Limited Data Request Information. Available online: https://hcai.ca.gov/data-and-reports/request-data/limited-data-request-information/ (accessed on 27 September 2023).
14. Centers for Disease Control and Prevention. International Classification of Diseases, Tenth Revision, Clinical Modification (ICD-10-CM). Available online: https://www.cdc.gov/nchs/icd/icd-10-cm.htm (accessed on 27 September 2023).
15. Agency for Healthcare Research and Quality. Healthcare Cost and Utilization Project User Support. Available online: https://hcup-us.ahrq.gov/db/vars/dispuniform/nisnote.jsp (accessed on 27 September 2023).
16. DeLaroche, A.M.; Rodean, J.; Aronson, P.L.; Fleegler, E.W.; Florin, T.A.; Goyal, M.; Hirsch, A.W.; Jain, S.; Kornblith, A.E.; Sills, M.R.; et al. Pediatric Emergency Department Visits at US Children's Hospitals During the COVID-19 Pandemic. *Pediatrics* **2021**, *147*, e2020039628. [CrossRef]
17. Birkmeyer, J.D.; Barnato, A.; Birkmeyer, N.; Bessler, R.; Skinner, J. The Impact of the COVID-19 Pandemic on Hospital Admissions in the United States. *Health Aff.* **2020**, *39*, 2010–2017. [CrossRef] [PubMed]
18. Nourazari, S.; Davis, S.R.; Granovsky, R.; Austin, R.; Straff, D.J.; Joseph, J.W.; Sanchez, L.D. Decreased Hospital Admissions through Emergency Departments during the COVID-19 Pandemic. *Am. J. Emerg. Med.* **2021**, *42*, 203–210. [CrossRef] [PubMed]
19. Bernardes, C.; Massano, J.; Freitas, A. Hospital Admissions 2000-2014: A Retrospective Analysis of 288 096 Events in Patients with Dementia. *Arch. Gerontol. Geriatr.* **2018**, *77*, 150–157. [CrossRef] [PubMed]
20. Sherzai, D.; Sherzai, A.; Lui, K.; Pan, D.; Chiou, D.; Bazargan, M.; Shaheen, M. The Association Between Diabetes and Dementia among Elderly Individuals: A Nationwide Inpatient Sample Analysis. *J. Geriatr. Psychiatry Neurol.* **2016**, *29*, 120–125. [CrossRef] [PubMed]
21. Fine, M.J.; Pratt, H.M.; Obrosky, D.S.; Lave, J.R.; McIntosh, L.J.; Singer, D.E.; Coley, C.M.; Kapoor, W.N. Relation between Length of Hospital Stay and Costs of Care for Patients with Community-Acquired Pneumonia. *Am. J. Med.* **2000**, *109*, 378–385. [CrossRef] [PubMed]
22. Lebrec, J.; Ascher-Svanum, H.; Chen, Y.; Reed, C.; Kahle-Wrobleski, K.; Hake, A.M.; Raskin, J.; Naderali, E.; Schuster, D.; Heine, R.J.; et al. Effect of Diabetes on Caregiver Burden in an Observational Study of Individuals with Alzheimer's Disease. *BMC Geriatr.* **2016**, *16*, 93. [CrossRef] [PubMed]
23. Freitas, A.; Silva-Costa, T.; Lopes, F.; Garcia-Lema, I.; Teixeira-Pinto, A.; Brazdil, P.; Costa-Pereira, A. Factors influencing hospital length of stay outliers. *BMC Health Serv. Res.* **2012**, *12*, 265. [CrossRef]
24. Lin, P.J.; Daly, A.T.; Olchanski, N.; Cohen, J.T.; Neumann, P.J.; Faul, J.D.; Fillit, H.M.; Freund, K.M. Dementia Diagnosis Disparities by Race and Ethnicity. *Med. Care* **2021**, *59*, 679–686. [CrossRef]
25. Haye, S.; Thunell, J.; Joyce, G.; Ferido, P.; Tysinger, B.; Jacobson, M.; Zissimopoulos, J. Estimates of diagnosed dementia prevalence and incidence among diverse beneficiaries in traditional Medicare and Medicare Advantage. *Alzheimer's Dement.* **2023**, *15*, e12472. [CrossRef]

26. Block, L.; Hovanes, M.; Gilmore-Bykovskyi, A.L. Written Discharge Communication of Diagnostic and Decision-Making Information for Persons Living with Dementia during Hospital to Skilled Nursing Facility Transitions. *Geriatr. Nurs.* **2022**, *45*, 215–222. [CrossRef]
27. Sadarangani, T.; Perissinotto, C.; Boafo, J.; Zhong, J.; Yu, G. Multimorbidity Patterns in Adult Day Health Center Clients with Dementia: A Latent Class Analysis. *BMC Geriatr.* **2022**, *22*, 514. [CrossRef] [PubMed]
28. Hodges, K.; Fox-Grage, W.; Tewarson, H.; The National Academy for State Health Policy. The Future of Aging Policy: A Snapshot of State Priorities. Available online: https://nashp.org/the-future-of-aging-policy-a-snapshot-of-state-priorities/ (accessed on 27 September 2023).
29. ElSayed, N.A.; Aleppo, G.; Aroda, V.R.; Bannuru, R.R.; Brown, F.M.; Bruemmer, D.; Collins, B.S.; Hilliard, M.E.; Isaacs, D.; Johnson, E.L.; et al. Classification and Diagnosis of Diabetes: Standards of Care in Diabetes-2023. *Diabetes Care* **2023**, *46* (Suppl. 1), S19–S40. [CrossRef] [PubMed]
30. Gaugler, J.E.; Borson, S.; Epps, F.; Shih, R.A.; Parker, L.J.; McGuire, L.C. The Intersection of Social Determinants of Health and Family Care of People Living with Alzheimer's Disease and Related Dementias: A Public Health Opportunity. *Alzheimers Dement.* **2023**, 1–10. [CrossRef] [PubMed]
31. Bauer, K.; Schwarzkopf, L.; Graessel, E.; Holle, R. A Claims Data-Based Comparison of Comorbidity in Individuals with and without Dementia. *BMC Geriatr.* **2014**, *14*, 10. [CrossRef] [PubMed]
32. Power, M.C.; Weuve, J.; Gagne, J.J.; McQueen, M.B.; Viswanathan, A.; Blacker, D. The Association between Blood Pressure and Incident Alzheimer Disease: A Systematic Review and Meta-Analysis. *Epidemiology* **2011**, *22*, 646–659. [CrossRef] [PubMed]
33. Sierra, C. Hypertension and the Risk of Dementia. *Front. Cardiovasc. Med.* **2020**, *7*, 5. [CrossRef] [PubMed]
34. Nagar, S.D.; Pemu, P.; Qian, J.; Boerwinkle, E.; Cicek, M.; Clark, C.R.; Cohn, E.; Gebo, K.; Loperena, R.; Mayo, K.; et al. Investigation of hypertension and type 2 diabetes as risk factors for dementia in the All of Us cohort. *Sci. Rep.* **2022**, *12*, 19797. [CrossRef] [PubMed]
35. Welsh, T.J.; Gladman, J.R.; Gordon, A.L. The treatment of hypertension in people with dementia: A systematic review of observational studies. *BMC Geriatr.* **2014**, *14*, 19. [CrossRef]
36. American Diabetes Association. Diabetes and High Blood Pressure. Diabetes and High Blood Pressure | ADA. (n.d.). Available online: https://diabetes.org/about-diabetes/complications/high-blood-pressure (accessed on 11 November 2023).
37. Centers for Disease Control and Prevention. National Diabetes Statistics Report Website. Available online: https://www.cdc.gov/diabetes/data/statistics-report/index.html (accessed on 11 November 2023).
38. Shinjyo, N.; Parkinson, J.; Bell, J.; Katsuno, T.; Bligh, A. Berberine for prevention of dementia associated with diabetes and its comorbidities: A systematic review. *J. Integr. Med.* **2020**, *18*, 125–151. [CrossRef]
39. Singhal, S.; Kumar, P.; Singh, S.; Saha, S.; Dey, A.B. Clinical Features and Outcomes of COVID-19 in Older Adults: A Systematic Review and Meta-Analysis. *BMC Geriatr.* **2021**, *21*, 321. [CrossRef]
40. Centers for Disease Control and Prevention. Underlying Medical Conditions Associated with Higher Risk for Severe COVID-19: Information for Healthcare Professionals. Available online: https://www.cdc.gov/coronavirus/2019-ncov/hcp/clinical-care/underlyingconditions.html (accessed on 27 September 2023).
41. Khunti, K.; Del Prato, S.; Mathieu, C.; Kahn, S.E.; Gabbay, R.A.; Buse, J.B. COVID-19, Hyperglycemia and New-Onset Diabetes. *Diabetes Care* **2021**, *44*, 2645–2655. [CrossRef] [PubMed]
42. Gasmi, A.; Peana, M.; Pivina, L.; Srinath, S.; Benahmed, A.G.; Semenova, Y.; Menzel, A.; Dadar, M.; Bjørklund, G. Interrelations between COVID-19 and Other Disorders. *Clin. Immunol.* **2021**, *224*, 108651. [CrossRef] [PubMed]
43. Kania, M.; Koń, B.; Kamiński, K.; Hohendorff, J.; Witek, P.; Klupa, T.; Malecki, M.T. Diabetes as a risk factor of death in hospitalized COVID-19 patients—An analysis of a National Hospitalization Database from Poland, 2020. *Front. Endocrinol.* **2023**, *14*, 1161637. [CrossRef] [PubMed]
44. Wang, Q.; Davis, P.B.; Gurney, M.E.; Xu, R. COVID-19 and dementia: Analyses of risk, disparity, and outcomes from electronic health records in the US. *Alzheimers Dement.* **2021**, *17*, 1297–1306. [CrossRef] [PubMed]
45. Dubey, S.; Das, S.; Ghosh, R.; Dubey, M.J.; Chakraborty, A.P.; Roy, D.; Dutta, A.; Santra, A.; Sengupta, S.; Benito-León, J. The Effects of SARS-CoV-2 Infection on the Cognitive Functioning of Patients with Pre-Existing Dementia. *J. Alzheimers Dis. Rep.* **2023**, *7*, 119–128. [CrossRef] [PubMed]
46. Lopez-de-Andres, A.; Jimenez-Garcia, R.; Zamorano-Leon, J.J.; Omaña-Palanco, R.; Carabantes-Alarcon, D.; Hernández-Barrera, V.; De Miguel-Diez, J.; Cuadrado-Corrales, N. Prevalence of Dementia among Patients Hosptialized with Type 2 Diabetes Mellitus in Spain, 2011-2020: Sex-Related Disparities and Impact of the COVID-19 Pandemic. *Int. J. Environ. Res.* **2023**, *20*, 4923. [CrossRef]
47. Einarson, T.R.; Acs, A.; Ludwig, C.; Panton, U.H. Prevalence of cardiovascular disease in type 2 diabetes: A systematic literature review of scientific evidence from across the world in 2007–2017. *Cardiovasc. Diabetol.* **2018**, *17*, 83. [CrossRef]
48. Alzheimer's Association. Alzheimer's and Multiple Chronic Conditions Fact Sheet. 2022. Available online: https://www.alz.org/media/Documents/alzheimers-and-multiple-chronic-conditions.pdf (accessed on 9 November 2023).
49. Bansal, M. Cardiovascular disease and COVID-19. *Diabetes Metab. Syndr. Clin. Res. Rev.* **2020**, *14*, 247–250. [CrossRef]
50. Clerkin, K.J.; Fried, J.A.; Raikhelkar, J.; Sayer, G.; Griffin, J.M.; Masoumi, A.; Jain, S.S.; Burkhoff, D.; Kumaraiah, D.; Rabbani, L.; et al. COVID-19 and Cardiovascular disease. *Circulation* **2020**, *141*, 1648–1655. [CrossRef]

51. Hessami, A.; Shamshirian, A.; Heydari, K.; Pourali, F.; Alizadeh-Navaei, R.; Moosazadeh, M.; Abrotan, S.; Shojaie, L.; Sedighi, S.; Shamshirian, D.; et al. Cardiovascular diseases burden in COVID-19: Systematic review and meta-analysis. *Am. J. Emerg. Med.* **2021**, *46*, 382–391. [CrossRef]
52. Alzheimer's Association. 2023 Alzheimer's Disease Facts and Figures. Available online: https://www.alz.org/media/documents/alzheimers-facts-and-figures.pdf (accessed on 27 September 2023).
53. Lin, J.; Thompson, T.J.; Cheng, Y.J.; Zhuo, X.; Zhang, P.; Gregg, E.; Rolka, D.B. Projection of the Future Diabetes Burden in the United States through 2060. *Popul. Health Metr.* **2018**, *16*, 9. [CrossRef] [PubMed]
54. Matthews, K.A.; Xu, W.; Gaglioti, A.H.; Holt, J.B.; Croft, J.B.; Mack, D.; McGuire, L.C. Racial and Ethnic Estimates of Alzheimer's Disease and Related Dementias in the United States (2015–2060) in Adults Aged ≥65 years. *Alzheimers Dement.* **2019**, *15*, 17–24. [CrossRef] [PubMed]
55. Hebert, L.E.; Weuve, J.; Scherr, P.A.; Evans, D.A. Alzheimer Disease in the United States (2010–2050) Estimated Using the 2010 Census. *Neurology* **2013**, *80*, 1778–1783. [CrossRef] [PubMed]
56. Braveman, P.; Arkin, E.; Proctor, D.; Kauh, T.; Holm, N.; Robert Wood Johnson Foundation. Systemic Racism and Health Equity. Available online: https://www.rwjf.org/en/insights/our-research/2021/12/systemic-racism-and-health-equity.html (accessed on 27 September 2023).
57. Yearby, R.; Clark, B.; Figueroa, J.F. Structural Racism in Historical and Modern US Health Care Policy. *Health Aff.* **2022**, *41*, 187–194. [CrossRef] [PubMed]
58. Bosisio, F.; Sterie, A.C.; Rubli Truchard, E.; Jox, R.J. Implementing Advance Care Planning in Early Dementia Care: Results and Insights from a Pilot Interventional Trial. *BMC Geriatr.* **2021**, *21*, 573. [CrossRef] [PubMed]
59. Dunning, T.L. Palliative and End-of-Life Care: Vital Aspects of Holistic Diabetes Care of Older People with Diabetes. *Diabetes Spectr.* **2020**, *33*, 246–254. [CrossRef] [PubMed]
60. Srikanth, V.; Sinclair, A.J.; Hill-Briggs, F.; Moran, C.; Biessels, G.J. Type 2 Diabetes and Cognitive Dysfunction-towards Effective Management of Both Comorbidities. *Lancet Diabetes Endocrinol.* **2020**, *8*, 535–545. [CrossRef] [PubMed]
61. Vuohijoki, A.; Mikkola, I.; Jokelainen, J.; Keinänen-Kiukaanniemi, S.; Winell, K.; Frittitta, L.; Timonen, M.; Hagnäs, M. Implementation of a Personalized Care Plan for Patients with Type 2 Diabetes is Associated with Improvements in Clinical Outcomes: An Observational Real-World Study. *J. Prim. Care Community Health* **2020**, *11*, 2150132720921700. [CrossRef]
62. Bunn, F.; Goodman, C.; Jones, P.R.; Russell, B.; Trivedi, D.; Sinclair, A.; Bayer, A.; Rait, G.; Rycroft-Malone, J.; Burton, C. Managing Diabetes in People with Dementia: A Realist Review. *Health Technol. Assess.* **2017**, *21*, 1–140. [CrossRef]
63. Kim, S.K.; Park, M. Effectiveness of Person-Centered Care on People with Dementia: A Systematic Review and Meta-Analysis. *Clin. Interv. Aging* **2017**, *12*, 381–397. [CrossRef]
64. Hopkins, R.; Shaver, K.; Weinstock, R.S. Management of Adults with Diabetes and Cognitive Problems. *Diabetes Spectr.* **2016**, *29*, 224–237. [CrossRef]
65. Fulmer, T.; Reuben, D.B.; Auerbach, J.; Fick, D.M.; Galambos, C.; Johnson, K.S. Actualizing Better Health and Health Care for Older Adults. *Health Aff.* **2021**, *40*, 219–225. [CrossRef]
66. Super, N. Three Trends Shaping the Politics of Aging in America. *Public Policy Aging Rep.* **2020**, *30*, 39–45. [CrossRef]
67. National Institute on Aging. National Institute on Aging: Strategic Directions for Research: 2020–2025. Available online: https://www.nia.nih.gov/about/aging-strategic-directions-research (accessed on 27 September 2023).

Disclaimer/Publisher's Note: The statements, opinions and data contained in all publications are solely those of the individual author(s) and contributor(s) and not of MDPI and/or the editor(s). MDPI and/or the editor(s) disclaim responsibility for any injury to people or property resulting from any ideas, methods, instructions or products referred to in the content.

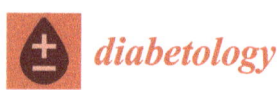 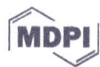

Article

Patients' Perspective on Barriers to Utilization of a Diabetic Retinopathy Screening Service

Bismark Owusu-Afriyie [1,2,*,†], Theresa Gende [1,2,†], Martin Tapilas [1], Nicholas Zimbare [1] and Jeffrey Kewande [1]

[1] Faculty of Medicine and Health Sciences, Divine Word University, Madang 511, Papua New Guinea; tgende@hollows.org.nz (T.G.); martintapilas@gmail.com (M.T.); niczimbare@gmail.com (N.Z.); jeffkewande@gmail.com (J.K.)
[2] The Fred Hollows Foundation NZ, Auckland 1010, New Zealand
* Correspondence: dr.bismarkoa@gmail.com; Tel.: +1-903-363-4122
† These authors contributed equally to this work.

Abstract: This study was conducted to determine the barriers to the utilization of diabetic retinopathy (DR) screening in Papua New Guinea (PNG). A list of patients booked for DR screening at Madang Provincial Hospital Eye Clinic (MPHEC) between January 2017 and December 2021 who had not been screened was retrieved, and the patients were invited to participate in the study. The data were collected using a structured questionnaire, and IBM Statistical Package for Social Sciences version 26 was used for the analysis. $p < 0.05$ was considered statistically significant. One hundred and twenty-nine patients (37.4%) did not attend DR screening for the period under study. The study response rate was 80.6%. The mean ± SD age of the respondents was 51.5 ± 10.9 years. The majority of the study respondents were female (62.5%), people living in rural settings (53.8%), and farmers (22.1%). Time constraints, poor knowledge about DR, and long waiting periods at the DR screening center were the main barriers to the uptake of DR screening. Compared to respondents in urban communities, those in rural settings were significantly concerned about cost ($p < 0.001$), travel distance to the MPHEC ($p < 0.001$), and poor information about DR screening ($p = 0.002$). More than half of the respondents (63.5%) had discontinued using pharmacotherapy for DM. There is a high rate of nonadherence to diabetes (DM) and DR treatment in PNG. There is a need for public health campaigns about DM and strategic DR screening at the community level in PNG and similar countries.

Keywords: barriers; diabetic retinopathy; diabetes; poor knowledge; cost; time constraints

Citation: Owusu-Afriyie, B.; Gende, T.; Tapilas, M.; Zimbare, N.; Kewande, J. Patients' Perspective on Barriers to Utilization of a Diabetic Retinopathy Screening Service. *Diabetology* 2023, 4, 393–405. https://doi.org/10.3390/diabetology4030033

Academic Editor: Peter Clifton

Received: 30 July 2023
Revised: 25 August 2023
Accepted: 5 September 2023
Published: 11 September 2023

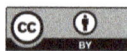

Copyright: © 2023 by the authors. Licensee MDPI, Basel, Switzerland. This article is an open access article distributed under the terms and conditions of the Creative Commons Attribution (CC BY) license (https://creativecommons.org/licenses/by/4.0/).

1. Introduction

Diabetic retinopathy (DR) is the most common complication of diabetes (DM) [1–3], and its main risk factors are disease duration, poor glycemic control, and hypertension [1]. The disease remains a clinical problem [4], and it is the leading cause of working age and adult-onset blindness in spite of improvements in diabetes care [2,5]. Thus, it is a great concern for people with diabetes and healthcare providers. Several years of research into the pathophysiology and management of DR have improved the understanding of the disease process [6–8]. In order to prevent sight loss from DR, all persons with diabetes are encouraged to undergo a comprehensive eye examination for the early detection and treatment of DR, herein referred to as DR screening.

DR is categorized into two main forms based on the clinical features of the disease, namely non-proliferative DR (NPDR) and proliferative DR (PDR) [9]. Cotton wool spots, retinal hemorrhages, retinal exudates, and microaneurysms are often the hallmark of NPDR. PDR is distinguished from NPDR by the presence of new blood vessels in the retina and/or iris (neovascularization). These new blood vessels are fragile and often cause further complications, such as vitreous hemorrhage. PDR, together with diabetic macular oedema, are the main causes of vision-threatening DR [10].

The low level of DR screening in Papua New Guinea (PNG), coupled with the growing prevalence of diabetes, is worrisome. Burnett et al. indicated in their study that more than three-quarters of the patients with known diabetes in the National Capital District of PNG never had an eye examination [11]. They further discovered that nearly half of those with diabetes had developed retinopathy and/or maculopathy [11]. While this low level of DR screening may be attributed to a lack of a national DR screening program in PNG, it is worth exploring the barriers to the utilization of DR screening in settings in the country where the service is available.

In 2007, the Madang Provincial Hospital Eye Clinic (MPHEC) implemented systematic DR screening for all people with diabetes to identify and treat sight-threatening retinopathy using the "Pacific Diabetes Retinal Screening, Grading and Management Guidelines" [12]. In this guideline, people with DM but no DR are expected to undertake annual retinal screening, while those with DR are scheduled for periodic screenings, depending on the clinical features and severity of the condition [12]. The MPHEC is one of the three centers in the country that offer DR screening, such as fundus photography and laser treatment. Ophthalmic clinicians and ophthalmologists in the country are trained to detect and refer DR cases to either the MPHEC or the other two centers at Port Moresby for further assessment and management. DR screening at the MPHEC is at no cost to the patients.

A recent finding indicated that 50% of all ophthalmic patients aged ≥30 years who visited the MPHEC in the first half of 2021 were either pre-diabetic or diabetic [13]; hence, it was paramount that they undergo DR screening. Despite the availability of the free retinal screening service at the facility, the uptake of the service has been very low, at an average of two patients per month for the years 2017 to 2021. It was therefore necessary to identify the reasons for the nonadherence to DR screening among patients who had records at the MPHEC.

This study explored the views of patients who had not yet attended DR screening or missed review appointments over a 5-year period. Our findings have the potential to direct policymakers to develop strategies to enhance the quality and uptake of DM and DR services in PNG and other similar countries.

2. Materials and Methods

2.1. Study Setting

The study was designed and conducted by using clinical records from the MPHEC. It was one of the three DR screening centers in PNG at the time of this study. The facility routinely screens patients aged ≥30 years for DM at no cost and, in addition, provides free DR services for walk-in and referred patients with diabetes (DM). Therefore, our study included patients from across the country, not just Madang Province. At the MPHEC and the other eye clinics, patients are first examined by an ophthalmologist or ophthalmic clinician before a recommendation is given for DR screening.

2.2. Study Design and Sampling Techniques

Purposive sampling was used in this descriptive cross-sectional study, as only DM and DR patients' records at the MPHEC were selected for the study.

2.3. Inclusion and Exclusion Criteria

The records of DM patients and the DR referral list of the MPHEC from January 2017 to December 2021 were reviewed, and those who had not yet undertaken DR screening or missed follow-up retinal screenings were selected. These patients were contacted via the phone, and standardized information about the identity of the researchers, the purpose of the study, the estimated time to complete the questionnaire, voluntary participation, privacy, confidentiality, and anonymity of the data to be collected was given to the patients before inviting them to participate in the study. The study excluded 20 patients who could not be reached, 4 patients who did not consent, 1 deceased patient, and records before January 2017 and after December 2021.

2.4. Data Collection Procedure

A structured questionnaire was designed based on similar studies [14–18] and used for this study (see Supplementary Material). It comprised four parts: the first part determined the respondents' sociodemographic data, the second portion evaluated the barriers directly related to the patients, the third aspect investigated service-related challenges, and the final set of questions inquired if the patients were on any diabetes treatment. The responses were rated on a 10-point scale, where 1 meant that it was not a barrier at all and 10 meant that it was a very strong barrier. Respondents were also given the opportunity to provide any further comments. Data collection was done during phone calls and in-person interactions when possible, and the respondents' responses were recorded by researchers M.T., J.K., and N.Z. Data was collected from June to October 2022.

2.5. Data Management and Analysis

The data were analyzed using IBM Statistical Package for Social Sciences (SPSS) version 26. Frequencies and percentages were used to summarize the categorical variables, while the continuous variables were summarized using means (±standard deviation) and medians (interquartile range). The Wilcoxon rank-sum test and Kruskal–Wallis test were used to determine associations, and Bonferroni correction was done for multiple comparisons. Statistical significance was established at $p < 0.05$.

3. Results

3.1. Sociodemographic Features of the Respondents

A total of 345 patients were listed in the DR screening and referral registers for the period under study, out of which 129 patients (37.4%) failed to undertake their first DR screenings or missed follow-up visits. Of this number, 104 patients participated in the study, giving a response rate of 80.6%. There were more female respondents (62.5%) than male. The age of the study respondents ranged from 24 to 75 years, with a mean of 51.5 ± 10.9 years. The majority of the respondents (53.8%) were from rural settings, and more than three-quarters of them were residents of Madang Province. Farming (22.1%) was the most common primary occupation among the respondents, and people with tertiary education (42.3%) were the highest respondents. The demographic characteristics of the study respondents are detailed in Table 1.

Table 1. Demographics of the study respondents.

Characteristics	Respondents; n (%)
Gender	
Male	39 (37.5)
Female	65 (62.5)
Residential Location	
Urban	48 (46.2)
Rural	56 (53.8)
Age Group (years)	
21–30	4 (3.8)
31–40	14 (13.5)
41–50	30 (28.8)
51–60	33 (31.7)
61–70	20 (19.2)
Above 70 years	3 (2.9)

Table 1. Cont.

Characteristics	Respondents; n (%)
Level of Education	
Primary	16 (15.4)
Secondary	34 (32.7)
Tertiary	44 (42.3)
No formal education	10 (9.6)
Residential Province	
Madang	89 (85.6)
Simbu	4 (3.8)
East New Britain	2 (1.9)
Milne Bay	2 (1.9)
Jiwaka	2 (1.9)
Others [a]	4 (3.8)
Not reported	1 (1.0)
Primary Occupation	
Farmer	23 (22.1)
Retail trader/self employed	14 (13.5)
Teacher/lecturer	12 (11.5)
Housewife	11 (10.6)
Manager/director	9 (8.7)
Health worker	7 (6.7)
Secretary	7 (6.7)
Others [b]	21 (20.2)
Expected Year of DR Screening	
2017	10 (9.6)
2018	15 (14.4)
2019	22 (21.2)
2020	44 (42.3)
2021	13 (12.5)
Category of Nonadherence	
First DR screening appointment	37 (35.6)
Follow-up visits/reviews	58 (55.8)
Taking Any Diabetes Treatment/Medication	
Yes	38 (36.5)
No	66 (63.5)
Diabetes Medication	
Metformin	27 (26.0)
Daonil	6 (5.8)
Herbs and traditional remedy	3 (2.9)
Insulin	1 (1.0)
Nifedipine	1 (1.0)

Table 1. *Cont.*

Characteristics	Respondents; n (%)
Reasons For Not Taking Diabetes Treatment	
No reason	32 (30.8)
Diet	21 (20.2)
Managing other comorbidity first	6 (5.8)
Poor access to a health facility	3 (2.9)
Financial constraint	2 (1.9)
Side effect of medication	1 (1.0)
Poor understanding of the treatment plan	1 (1.0)

[a] East Sepik—1; Enga—1; Morobe—1; Eastern Highlands—1. [b] Musician—2; Retired—4; Sailor—1; Air traffic staff—1; Customer care representative—5; Electrician—1; Carpenter—1; Security person—3; Unemployed—2; Clergy—1.

3.2. Personal Barriers

The majority of respondents indicated that time constraints (86.5%) was a barrier to their uptake of DR screenings. In addition, more than half of the respondents considered poor knowledge about DR, cost, good vision in the fellow eye, their eye problem not being a serious issue, the need for a guardian, no reminders about screening appointments, and the asymptomatic nature of their conditions as their personal reasons for not attending DR screenings. The details are shown in Table 2.

Table 2. Reported barriers to DR screening.

Personal Barriers	Respondents; n (%)
Insufficient income or cost	54 (51.9)
Good vision in the fellow eye	58 (55.8)
Eye problem is not serious enough	73 (70.2)
Time constraints or other priorities	90 (86.5)
No escort or guardian to help	56 (53.8)
Culture/traditional beliefs	34 (32.7)
Forgot or no reminder	62 (59.6)
No symptoms	57 (54.8)
Poor knowledge about DR	80 (76.9)
Prefer to use alternative service	42 (40.3)
Service-related Barriers	**Respondents; n (%)**
Not well informed that I need DR screening	68 (65.4)
Do not know where to get services	36 (34.6)
Eye/screening center is too far	58 (55.8)
Long waiting time at eye/screening center	81 (77.9)
Low quality service by clinicians	32 (30.8)
Unfriendly staff at eye/screening center	33 (31.7)
Fear of procedure complications	78 (75.0)
Lack of trust in healthcare institutions	38 (36.5)

Among all the respondents, the most important personal barriers to DR screenings were time constraints (median (IQR) = 7/10 (9/10–3/10)) and poor knowledge about DR (median (IQR) = 5/10 (9/10–2/10)). Overall, culture and traditional beliefs and the use of an alternative treatment did not appear to be hindrances to DR screening services among the respondents (each median (IQR) = 1/10 (2/10–1/10)). The details are shown in Figure 1.

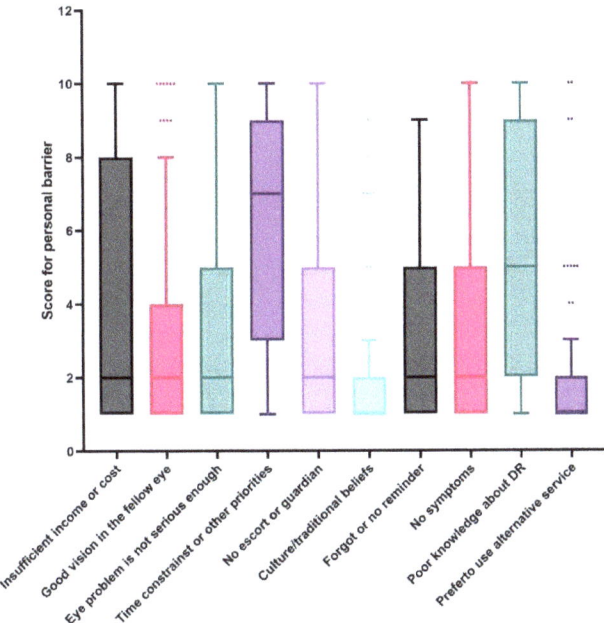

Figure 1. General personal barriers to diabetic retinopathy screening in Madang District. Responses were rated from 1 (not a barrier) to 10 (a very strong barrier). Center lines indicate the medians; box limits indicate the 25th and 75th percentiles; whiskers extend 1.5 times the interquartile range. Dots indicate outliers.

Respondents from rural settings more often indicated that insufficient income or cost (median (IQR) = 8/10 (10/10–1/10)), having other priorities that demanded their time (median (IQR) = 8/10 (9/10–4.3/10)), and poor knowledge about DR (median (IQR) = 7/10 (9/10–2/10)) were the main personal challenges to DR screenings (Figure 2A). Similarly, the most important personal barriers to DR screening among respondents in urban communities were time constraints (median (IQR) = 5/10 (8/10–2/10)) and poor knowledge about DR (median (IQR) = 3/10 (8/10–1/10)). The details are shown in Figure 2A. Respondents from rural settings reported cost ($p < 0.001$), having good vision in the fellow eye ($p = 0.040$), time constraints ($p = 0.016$), poor knowledge about DR ($p = 0.007$), the need for a guardian ($p < 0.001$), and reminders ($p = 0.001$) as significant barriers compared to respondents from urban settings (Figure 2A).

There was no statistically significant difference in the responses from males and females (Figure 2B). From Figure 2C, respondents without formal education significantly considered their eye problems as not being serious enough compared to respondents with secondary ($p = 0.013$) and tertiary educations ($p = 0.029$).

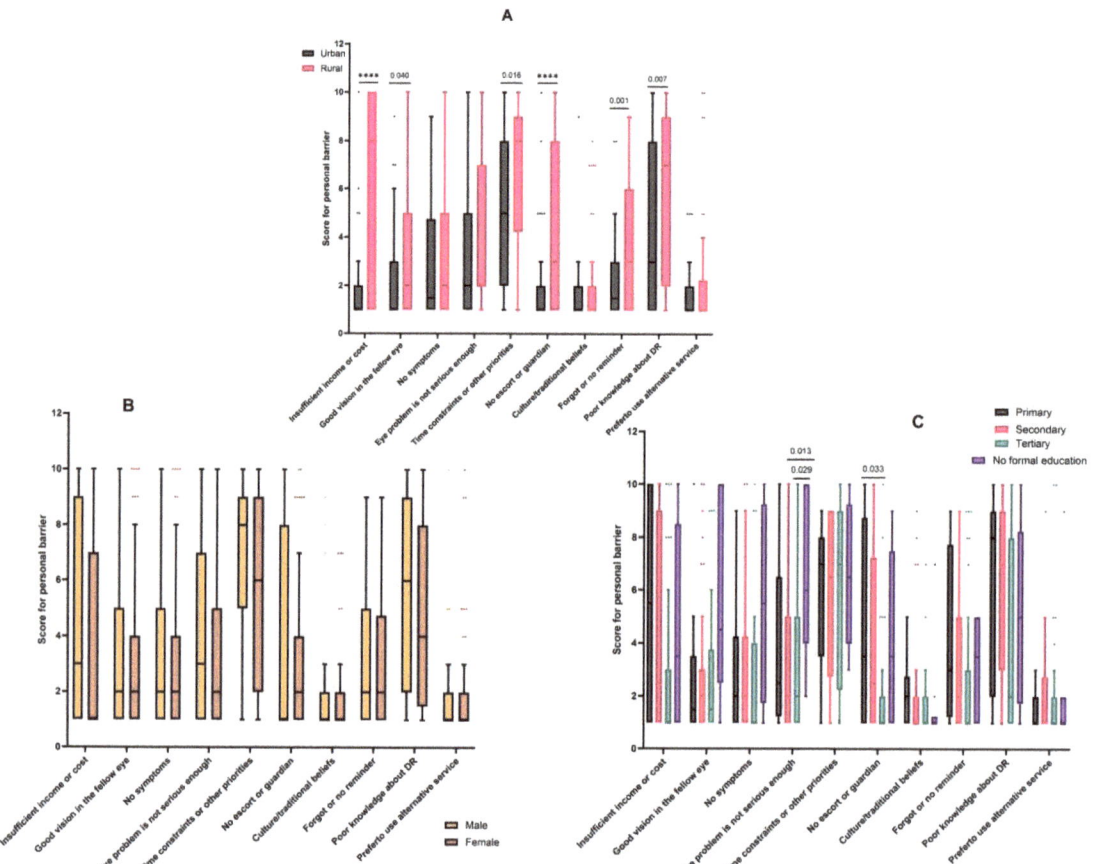

Figure 2. Demographic analysis of personal barriers to DR screening services in Madang District. Responses were rated from 1 (not a barrier) to 10 (a very strong barrier). Center lines indicate the medians; box limits indicate the 25th and 75th percentiles; whiskers extend 1.5 times the interquartile range. Dots indicate outliers. Comparisons were determined using the Wilcoxon rank-sum test (**A**,**B**) and Kruskal–Wallis test with Bonferroni correction (**C**). Statistically significant values are reported on the graphs. **** $p < 0.001$.

3.3. Service-Related Barriers

At the service level, the majority of the respondents were concerned about long waiting times at the eye screening center (77.9%), fear of procedure complications (75.0%), not being well informed about DR screening (65.4%), and the distant location of the screening center (55.8%) (see Table 2). The main service-related barriers to the uptake of DR screening among all the respondents were the long waiting periods at the eye center (median (IQR) = 5/10 (9/10–2/10)), not being well informed about DR screening (median (IQR) = 3/10 (5.8/10–1/10)), and a fear of procedure complications (median (IQR) = 3/10(3/10–1.3/10)). Further details are shown in Figure 3A.

Respondents from rural communities were more concerned about the long waiting times at the screening center (median (IQR) = 8/10 (9/10–3/10)) and proximity (median (IQR) = 8/10(10/10–1.25/10)). Respondents from urban settings also showed increased concern about the long waiting periods at the screening center (median (IQR) = 5/10 (9/10–1/10)). Barriers such as not being well informed that the respondents needed DR screening and the long-distance location of the screening center were significantly reported by respondents in rural settings compared to their urban counterparts ($p = 0.002$ and <0.001, respectively). These are highlighted in Figure 3B. Similar responses were reported by respondents with secondary and tertiary educations ($p = 0.048$ and 00.46, respectively; Figure 3D). The responses from male and female respondents were comparable (Figure 3C); however, the female respondents were significantly concerned about unfriendly staff at the screening center ($p = 0.006$).

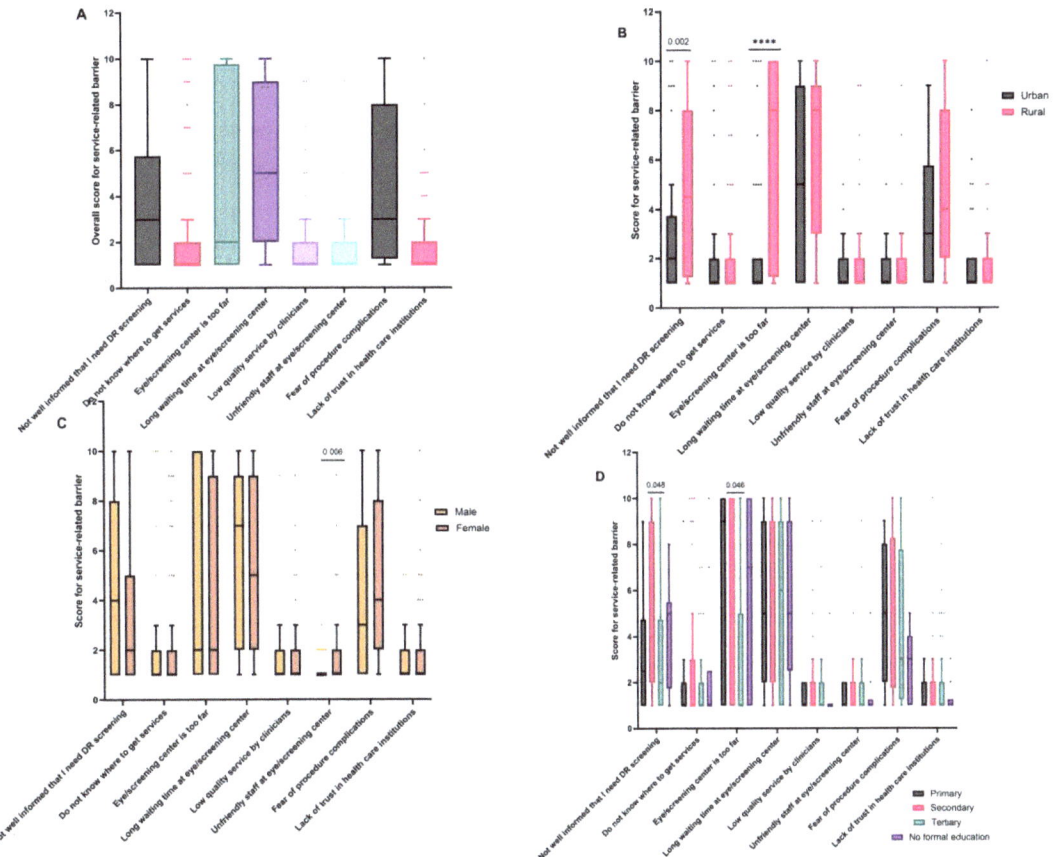

Figure 3. Analysis of the service-related barriers to DR screening services in Madang District. The responses were rated from 1 (not a barrier) to 10 (a very strong barrier). The overall service-related barriers were analyzed (**A**), and comparisons were determined using Wilcoxon rank-sum test (**B**,**C**) and Kruskal–Wallis test with Bonferroni correction (**D**). Center lines indicate the medians; box limits indicate the 25th and 75th percentiles; whiskers extend 1.5 times the interquartile range. Dots indicate outliers. Statistically significant values are reported on the graphs. **** $p < 0.001$.

4. Discussion

There is a rise in the global prevalence of DM, and current projections indicate that 1.3 billion people will have DM by the year 2050 [19]. This will have significant implications for the eye health sector due to the effect and complications of DM on the eyes. Patients with DM may not be aware of its damaging effects on their eyes until the onset of visual symptoms; by which time, any sight loss is irreversible. However, sight loss caused by complications of DM can be prevented by timely and effective interventions, such as regular DR screening and early treatment [15]. An effective screening and management program requires that patients and their caregivers are willing to actively adhere to treatment protocols. This study aimed to understand the barriers influencing DR screening nonattendance at one of the three DR screening centers in PNG and propose measures to address these challenges.

The World Health Organization recently recommended that countries should monitor the proportion of people with DM attending DR screening appointments, preferably by using data from health facilities [20]. DR screening is at no cost to patients who visit the MPHEC, but a substantial proportion of DM patients (37.4%) did not attend DR screening during the period under review. Suboptimal adherence to DR screening is not unique to this setting and other developing countries. In Australia, retinal screening coverage among people with DM remains a challenge in spite of Medicare benefits that include non-mydriatic fundus photography due to other barriers, such as time constraints, the cost of retinal cameras, and a lack of expertise in delivering DR services [16]. It is well established that DR is the most significant cause of visual impairment and blindness among adults and the working age population [21,22]. In this study, the average age of the respondents was 51.5 ± 10.9 years, similar to a study in Saudi Arabia that reported an average age of 54.0 years [14]. All these data suggest that both developed and developing economies are at risk of losing a productive workforce if measures are not put in place to strengthen the adherence to DR screening programs.

Irrespective of the sociodemographic characteristics of the respondents, poor knowledge about DR, time constraints, and long waiting periods at the eye center were the main influencers associated with nonadherence to DR screening. A recent study reported that the majority of ophthalmic patients in Madang Province depend on health facilities for information about DM and DR [23]. Taken together with the outcomes of the current study, the two studies support a need for public education on DM and its complications in PNG and similar settings. An effective public health education about the complications of DM, effects of DR, and the benefits of timely and regular DR screening among persons with DM could reduce the burden of sight-threatening DR in PNG. This is especially important among respondents in rural communities and those with less than a secondary level of education.

High proportions of the patients who failed to attend DR screening in this study were female (62.5%), people living in rural communities (53.8%), and farmers (22.1%). Cost (such as for transport, accommodations, and food) was a major barrier to DR screening among respondents living in rural settings. Respondents from rural settings were also more often concerned about the distant location of the DR screening center from their homes. Socioeconomic deprivation is a major risk for nonattendance of DR screenings even in developed countries such as the United States of America, the United Kingdom, and Saudi Arabia [15]. Xiao et al. suggested that DR outreach screenings in rural communities in China are more reliable in reaching women, older populations, and less-educated individuals compared to passive case detection in hospitals and referral centers [24]. Therefore, a mobile DR screening program is an effective strategy that could be adopted in PNG to meet the population demands and enhance the uptake of DR services.

With the advancements in technology and teleophthalmology and the easy access to smartphones, stakeholders of eye care in PNG could consider implementing smartphone-based and/or portable handheld fundus imaging in rural and resource-constrained communities. Although this strategy may not replace conventional fundus photography at present, reports indicate that it is cost effective and has high accuracy at detecting sight-threatening DR [25–28]. This can increase the accessibility to DR screening services and minimize the long waiting periods at the screening center. In addition, the government and non-governmental organizations in PNG could consider subsidizing the cost of conventional retinal cameras to make them readily available in primary and secondary health care facilities and plan towards a national DR screening program. These proposed measures would require that clinicians in these facilities are well trained to use the fundus cameras for effective DR screening, a greater investment into the eye health workforce, and integration with the diabetes sector.

In many resource-constrained settings, clinicians rely on microvascular changes observed via ophthalmoscopy and/or retinal photography to diagnose, grade, and monitor the treatment of DR. However, the available data have shown that DR is not only a vascular disease but also shows neurodegenerative dysfunction [9]. Neural changes may occur before microvascular changes and visual defects are detected in the clinic. For example, in their quest to find biomarkers for the early diagnosis of DR, Harrison et al. found that multifocal electroretinogram was a powerful tool to predict the development of DR among persons with DM but no retinopathy [29]. Therefore, it is important that health care service providers and clinicians explore diagnostic techniques that examine both neural and vascular changes for the efficient and accurate diagnosis of DM and DR.

At present, binocular indirect ophthalmoscopy and fundus photography are the tests performed to detect DR among patients reporting to the MPHEC. Evidence suggests that other techniques such as electroretinogram [29,30], optical coherence tomography (OCT), and OCT angiography [10,30–34] provide additional key features and information for the early and improved diagnosis of DM and DR, as well as monitoring the treatments. These retinal imaging tools could be explored by DR screening centers such as the MPHEC, albeit this would require the training of clinicians and financial investments in the technologies, as previously noted above.

The study further investigated whether the study respondents were still taking their DM medications. Unexpectedly, two-thirds of them (63.5%) were not on any medication; out of which, 32 (30.8%) had no reason for refusing treatment, while 21 (20.2%) reported that they were managing their condition with diet instead of drugs. Despite the fact that there is no complete cure for DM at the time of this study, patient-centered care [35–37] and adherence to pharmacotherapy and lifestyle changes are extremely valuable in reducing hyperglycemia and, hence, complications of DM, including DR [36,38–40]. This study remarks the need for a future study to identify the barriers and influencers of nonadherence to DM treatment in PNG to reduce the burden of DM and its complications in the country. In addition, since blood glucose levels fluctuate [41], we recommend that healthcare facilities that provide DM and DR screening services such as the MPHEC could include the measurement of glycated hemoglobin (HbA1c) in their tests. HbA1c measures the blood glucose history over the previous two to three months and therefore provides a better understanding of a glycemic control compared to only a fasting or random blood glucose measurement [42,43]. Hence, it is a better predictor of DM and its complications.

The current evidence provides insight into DR screening services in PNG, but the findings are focused only on patients who were identified by or referred to the MPHEC during the 5-year period. Further study is necessary to detect the barriers to DM and DR care across communities in PNG and at the national level and implement appropriate interventions.

5. Conclusions

Ophthalmic clinicians and ophthalmologists in PNG are trained to examine the retina and refer patients for appropriate treatment based on the Pacific Diabetes Retinal Screening, Grading and Management Guidelines, yet a large proportion of persons with DM remain unscreened. This study identified time constraints, cost, poor knowledge about DR, long waiting times, and long travel distance to the DR screening center as the main barriers to the uptake of DR screening services. Several enabling strategies have been proposed in this study to increase the access to and adherence to DR screening at the MPHEC and across PNG.

Supplementary Materials: The following supporting information can be downloaded at https://www.mdpi.com/article/10.3390/diabetology4030033/s1: File S1: the questionnaire.

Author Contributions: Conceptualization, B.O.-A., T.G., M.T., N.Z. and J.K.; Data curation, B.O.-A., T.G., M.T., N.Z. and J.K.; Formal analysis, B.O.-A., T.G., M.T., N.Z. and J.K.; Methodology, B.O.-A., T.G., M.T., N.Z. and J.K.; Resources, B.O.-A., T.G., M.T., N.Z. and J.K.; Writing—original draft, B.O.-A.,

T.G., M.T., N.Z. and J.K.; Writing—review and editing, B.O.-A., T.G., M.T., N.Z. and J.K. All authors have read and agreed to the published version of the manuscript.

Funding: This research received no external funding, and the APC was funded by The Fred Hollows Foundation, NZ.

Institutional Review Board Statement: The study was conducted according to the guidelines of the Declaration of Helsinki and approved by The Faculty of Medicine and Health Sciences Research Committee of Divine Word University (approval number FRC/MHS/58-22 on 10 June 2022). Permission was granted by the management of the MPHEC in order to access the patients' records and contact details.

Informed Consent Statement: Informed consent was obtained from all subjects involved in the study. No personally identifiable information was collected as part of the study, and participation was voluntary and confidential.

Data Availability Statement: The data presented in this study are available upon request from the corresponding author. The data are not publicly available due to the use of a questionnaire for data collection.

Acknowledgments: We are grateful to the management of the MPHEC for granting us access to the DR screening lists and Carmilla Yawi for helping us to retrieve the lists. We thank The Fred Hollows Foundation, NZ for funding the APC.

Conflicts of Interest: The authors declare no conflict of interest.

References

1. Simó-Servat, O.; Hernández, C.; Simó, R. Diabetic Retinopathy in the Context of Patients with Diabetes. *Ophthalmic Res.* **2019**, *62*, 211–217. [CrossRef]
2. Jenkins, A.J.; Joglekar, M.V.; Hardikar, A.A.; Keech, A.C.; O'Neal, D.N.; Januszewski, A.S. Biomarkers in diabetic retinopathy. *Rev. Diabet. Stud.* **2015**, *12*, 159–195. [CrossRef] [PubMed]
3. Wang, W.; Lo, A.C.Y. Diabetic retinopathy: Pathophysiology and treatments. *Int. J. Mol. Sci.* **2018**, *19*, 1816. [CrossRef]
4. Hammes, H.P. Diabetic retinopathy: Hyperglycaemia, oxidative stress and beyond. *Diabetologia* **2018**, *61*, 29–38. [CrossRef]
5. Kang, Q.; Yang, C. Oxidative stress and diabetic retinopathy: Molecular mechanisms, pathogenetic role and therapeutic implications. *Redox Biol.* **2020**, *37*, 101799. [CrossRef] [PubMed]
6. Heng, L.Z.; Comyn, O.; Peto, T.; Tadros, C.; Ng, E.; Sivaprasad, S.; Hykin, P.G. Diabetic retinopathy: Pathogenesis, clinical grading, management and future developments. *Diabet. Med.* **2013**, *30*, 640–650. [CrossRef]
7. Rodríguez, M.L.; Pérez, S.; Mena-Mollá, S.; Desco, M.C.; Ortega, Á.L. Oxidative Stress and Microvascular Alterations in Diabetic Retinopathy: Future Therapies. *Oxid. Med. Cell. Longev.* **2019**, *2019*, 4940825. [CrossRef]
8. Al Ghamdi, A.H. Clinical Predictors of Diabetic Retinopathy Progression; A Systematic Review. *Curr. Diabetes Rev.* **2019**, *16*, 242–247. [CrossRef]
9. Chen, X.D.; Gardner, T.W. A critical review: Psychophysical assessments of diabetic retinopathy. *Surv. Ophthalmol.* **2021**, *66*, 213–230. [CrossRef]
10. Jampol, L.M.; Glassman, A.R.; Sun, J. Evaluation and Care of Patients with Diabetic Retinopathy. *N. Engl. J. Med.* **2020**, *382*, 1629–1637. [CrossRef]
11. Burnett, A.; Lee, L.; D'Esposito, F.; Wabulembo, G.; Cama, A.; Guldan, G.; Nelisse, M.; Koim, S.P.; Keys, D.; Poffley, A.J.; et al. Rapid assessment of avoidable blindness and diabetic retinopathy in people aged 50 years and older in the National Capital District of Papua New Guinea. *Br. J. Ophthalmol.* **2019**, *103*, 743–747. [CrossRef] [PubMed]
12. Pacific Eye Institute. *Diabetes Retinal Screening, Grading and Management Guidelines for Use in Pacific Island Nations, 2010*; Diabetes Work Group, Fred Hollows Found Pacific Eye Institute: Auckland, New Zealand, 2010; pp. 1–37. Available online: https://www.worlddiabetesfoundation.org/sites/default/files/WDF08-386%20Pacific%20Island%20Ret%20Screen%20Guidelines.pdf (accessed on 20 July 2023).
13. Owusu-afriyie, B.; Baimur, I.; Gende, T.; Baia, T. Prevalence of Risk Factors of Retinal Diseases among Patients in Madang Province, Papua New Guinea. *Int. J. Clin. Pract.* **2022**, *2022*, 6120908. [CrossRef]
14. Alwazae, M.; Al Adel, F.; Alhumud, A.; Almutairi, A.; Alhumidan, A.; Elmorshedy, H. Barriers for Adherence to Diabetic Retinopathy Screening among Saudi Adults. *Cureus* **2019**, *11*, e6454. [CrossRef] [PubMed]
15. Kashim, R.M.; Newton, P.; Ojo, O. Diabetic Retinopathy Screening: A Systematic Review on Patients' Non-Attendance. *Int. J. Environ. Res. Public. Health* **2018**, *15*, 157. [CrossRef] [PubMed]
16. Watson, M.J.G.; McCluskey, P.J.; Grigg, J.R.; Kanagasingam, Y.; Daire, J.; Estai, M. Barriers and facilitators to diabetic retinopathy screening within Australian primary care. *BMC Fam. Pract.* **2021**, *22*, 239. [CrossRef] [PubMed]
17. Bruggeman, B.; Zimmerman, C.; LaPorte, A.; Stalvey, M.; Filipp, S.L.; Gurka, M.J.; Silverstein, J.H.; Jacobsen, L.M. Barriers to retinopathy screening in youth and young adults with type 1 diabetes. *Pediatr. Diabetes* **2021**, *22*, 469–473. [CrossRef] [PubMed]

18. Fairless, E.; Nwanyanwu, K. Barriers to and Facilitators of Diabetic Retinopathy Screening Utilization in a High-Risk Population. *J. Racial Ethn. Health Disparities* **2019**, *6*, 1244–1249. [CrossRef] [PubMed]
19. Ong, K.L.; Stafford, L.K.; McLaughlin, S.A.; Boyko, E.J.; Vollset, S.E.; Smith, A.E.; Dalton, B.E.; Duprey, J.; Cruz, J.A.; Hagins, H.; et al. Global, regional, and national burden of diabetes from 1990 to 2021, with projections of prevalence to 2050: A systematic analysis for the Global Burden of Disease Study 2021. *Lancet* **2023**, *402*, 203–234. [CrossRef]
20. World Health Organization. Eye Care Indicator Menu (ECIM): A Tool for Monitoring Strategies and Actions for Eye Care Provision. 2022. Available online: http://apps.who.int/ (accessed on 21 July 2023).
21. Teo, Z.L.; Tham, Y.C.; Yu, M.; Chee, M.L.; Rim, T.H.; Cheung, N.; Bikbov, M.M.; Wang, Y.X.; Tang, Y.; Lu, Y.; et al. Global Prevalence of Diabetic Retinopathy and Projection of Burden through 2045: Systematic Review and Meta-analysis. *Ophthalmology* **2021**, *128*, 1580–1591. [CrossRef]
22. Sabanayagam, C.; Banu, R.; Chee, M.L.; Lee, R.; Wang, Y.X.; Tan, G.; Jonas, J.B.; Lamoureux, E.L.; Cheng, C.-Y.; Klein, B.E.K.; et al. Incidence and progression of diabetic retinopathy: A systematic review. *Lancet Diabetes Endocrinol.* **2019**, *7*, 140–149. [CrossRef]
23. Owusu-Afriyie, B.; Caleb, A.; Kube, L.; Gende, T. Knowledge and Awareness of Diabetes and Diabetic Retinopathy among Patients Seeking Eye Care Services in Madang Province, Papua New Guinea. *J. Ophthalmol.* **2022**, *2022*, 7674928. [CrossRef]
24. Xiao, B.; Mercer, G.D.; Jin, L.; Lee, H.L.; Chen, T.; Wang, Y.; Liu, Y.; Denniston, A.K.; Egan, C.A.; Li, J.; et al. Outreach screening to address demographic and economic barriers to diabetic retinopathy care in rural China. *PLoS ONE* **2022**, *17*, e0266380. [CrossRef] [PubMed]
25. Malerbi, F.K.; Andrade, R.E.; Morales, P.H.; Stuchi, J.A.; Lencione, D.; de Paulo, J.V.; Carvalho, M.P.; Nunes, F.S.; Rocha, R.M.; Ferraz, D.A.; et al. Diabetic Retinopathy Screening Using Artificial Intelligence and Handheld Smartphone-Based Retinal Camera. *J. Diabetes Sci. Technol.* **2022**, *16*, 716–723. [CrossRef] [PubMed]
26. Rajalakshmi, R.; Arulmalar, S.; Usha, M.; Prathiba, V.; Kareemuddin, K.S.; Anjana, R.M.; Mohan, V. Validation of smartphone based retinal photography for diabetic retinopathy screening. *PLoS ONE* **2015**, *10*, e0138285. [CrossRef] [PubMed]
27. Tan, C.H.; Kyaw, B.M.; Smith, H.; Tan, C.S.; Car, L.T. Use of Smartphones to Detect Diabetic Retinopathy: Scoping Review and Meta-Analysis of Diagnostic Test Accuracy Studies. *J. Med. Internet Res.* **2020**, *22*, e16658. [CrossRef] [PubMed]
28. Bilong, Y.; Katte, J.C.; Koki, G.; Kagmeni, G.; Obama, O.P.N.; Fofe, H.R.N.; Mvilongo, C.; Nkengfack, O.; Bimbai, A.M.; Sobngwi, E.; et al. Validation of smartphone-based retinal photography for diabetic retinopathy screening. *Ophthalmic Surg. Lasers Imaging Retin.* **2019**, *50*, S18–S22. [CrossRef] [PubMed]
29. Harrison, W.W.; Bearse, M.A.; Ng, J.S.; Jewell, N.P.; Barez, S.; Burger, D.; Schneck, M.E.; Adams, A.J. Multifocal electroretinograms predict onset of diabetic retinopathy in adult patients with diabetes. *Investig. Ophthalmol. Vis. Sci.* **2011**, *52*, 772–777. [CrossRef]
30. Zagst, A.J.; Smith, J.D.; Wang, R.; Harrison, W.W. Foveal avascular zone size and mfERG metrics in diabetes and prediabetes: A pilot study of the relationship between structure and function. *Doc. Ophthalmol.* **2023**, *147*, 99–107. [CrossRef]
31. Russell, J.F.; Al-khersan, H.; Shi, Y.; Scott, N.L.; Hinkle, J.W.; Fan, K.C.; Lyu, C.; Feuer, W.J.; Gregori, G.; Rosenfeld, P.J. Retinal Non-Perfusion in Proliferative Diabetic Retinopathy Before and After Panretinal Photocoagulation Assessed by Wide Field OCT Angiography. *Am. J. Ophthalmol.* **2020**, *213*, 177–185. [CrossRef]
32. Kyei, S.; Asare, F.A.; Assan, J.K.; Zaabaar, E.; Assiamah, F.; Obeng, E.O.; Asiedu, K. Efficacy of intravitreal bevacizumab on diabetic macular oedema in an African population. *Ir. J. Med. Sci.* **2023**. [CrossRef]
33. Sun, Z.; Yang, D.; Tang, Z.; Ng, D.S.; Cheung, C.Y. Optical coherence tomography angiography in diabetic retinopathy: An updated review. *Eye* **2021**, *35*, 149–161. [CrossRef]
34. Chua, J.; Sim, R.; Tan, B.; Wong, D.; Yao, X.; Liu, X.; Ting, D.S.W.; Schmidl, D.; Ang, M.; Garhöfer, G.; et al. Optical coherence tomography angiography in diabetes and diabetic retinopathy. *J. Clin. Med.* **2020**, *9*, 1723. [CrossRef] [PubMed]
35. Davies, M.J.; D'Alessio, D.A.; Fradkin, J.; Kernan, W.N.; Mathieu, C.; Mingrone, G.; Rossing, P.; Tsapas, A.; Wexler, D.J.; Buse, J.B. Management of hyperglycaemia in type 2 diabetes, 2018. A consensus report by the American Diabetes Association (ADA) and the European Association for the Study of Diabetes (EASD). *Diabetologia* **2018**, *61*, 2461–2498. [CrossRef]
36. Davies, M.J.; Aroda, V.R.; Collins, B.S.; Gabbay, R.A.; Green, J.; Maruthur, N.M.; Rosas, S.E.; Del Prato, S.; Mathieu, C.; Mingrone, G.; et al. Management of hyperglycaemia in type 2 diabetes, 2022. A consensus report by the American Diabetes Association (ADA) and the European Association for the Study of Diabetes (EASD). *Diabetologia* **2022**, *65*, 1925–1966. [CrossRef] [PubMed]
37. American Diabetes Association. Glycemic targets: Standards of medical care in diabetes. *Diabetes Care* **2022**, *42*, S61–S70.
38. Agrawal, L.; Azad, N.; Bahn, G.D.; Reaven, P.D.; Hayward, R.A.; Reda, D.J.; Emanuele, N.V.; Abraira, C.; Duckworth, W.C.; Hayden, C.T.; et al. Intensive glycemic control improves long-term renal outcomes in type 2 diabetes in the veterans affairs diabetes trial (VADT). *Diabetes Care* **2019**, *42*, E181–E182. [CrossRef] [PubMed]
39. Sun, S.; Hisland, L.; Grenet, G.; Gueyffier, F.; Cornu, C.; Jaafari, N.; Boussageon, R. Reappraisal of the efficacy of intensive glycaemic control on microvascular complications in patients with type 2 diabetes: A meta-analysis of randomised control-trials. *Therapies* **2022**, *77*, 413–423. [CrossRef]
40. Xu, H.; Li, X.; Adams, H.; Kubena, K.; Guo, S. Etiology of metabolic syndrome and dietary intervention. *Int. J. Mol. Sci.* **2019**, *20*, 128. [CrossRef]
41. Umpierrez, G.E.; PKovatchev, B. Glycemic Variability: How to Measure and Its Clinical Implication for Type 2 Diabetes. *Am. J. Med. Sci.* **2018**, *356*, 518–527. [CrossRef]

42. Sherwani, S.I.; Khan, H.A.; Ekhzaimy, A.; Masood, A.; Sakharkar, M.K. Significance of HbA1c test in diagnosis and prognosis of diabetic patients. *Biomark. Insights* **2016**, *11*, 95–104. [CrossRef]
43. Martinez, M.; Santamarina, J.; Pavesi, A.; Musso, C.; Umpierrez, G.E. Glycemic variability and cardiovascular disease in patients with type 2 diabetes. *BMJ Open Diabetes Res. Care* **2021**, *9*, e002032. [CrossRef]

Disclaimer/Publisher's Note: The statements, opinions and data contained in all publications are solely those of the individual author(s) and contributor(s) and not of MDPI and/or the editor(s). MDPI and/or the editor(s) disclaim responsibility for any injury to people or property resulting from any ideas, methods, instructions or products referred to in the content.

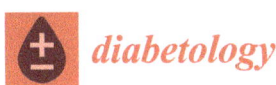

Review

Sexual Dysfunction in Female Patients with Type 2 Diabetes Mellitus—Sneak Peek on an Important Quality of Life Determinant

Marija Rogoznica [1,*], Dražen Perica [2], Barbara Borovac [3], Andrej Belančić [4,5] and Martina Matovinović [6]

1. Department of Physical Medicine, Rehabilitation and Rheumatology, Thalassotherapia Opatija, Maršala Tita 188, 51410 Opatija, Croatia
2. Department of Internal Medicine, Division of Metabolic Diseases, University Hospital Center Zagreb, Kišpatićeva 12, 10000 Zagreb, Croatia; drazen.perica1@gmail.com
3. Department of Gynecology and Obstetrics, Clinical Hospital Centre Rijeka, Krešimirova 42, 51000 Rijeka, Croatia; borovacbarbara@gmail.com
4. Department of Clinical Pharmacology, Clinical Hospital Centre Rijeka, Krešimirova 42, 51000 Rijeka, Croatia; a.belancic93@gmail.com or andrej.belancic@uniri.hr
5. Department of Basic and Clinical Pharmacology with Toxicology, Faculty of Medicine, University of Rijeka, Braće Branchetta 20, 51000 Rijeka, Croatia
6. Department of Internal Medicine, Division of Endocrinology, University Hospital Center Zagreb, Kišpatićeva 12, 10000 Zagreb, Croatia; martina_10000@yahoo.com
* Correspondence: marija.rogoznica@tto.hr

Abstract: Type 2 diabetes mellitus (T2DM) is a multisystemic disease with a high global burden and chronic complications. Sexual dysfunction (SD) in patients with T2DM is an often-overlooked complication, despite its high impact on quality of life (QoL). Female sexual disorders can affect women of reproductive age as well as menopausal women. Proposed mechanisms are intertwining a variety of physiological, neurological, vascular, hormonal, and psychological variables. The impairment of sexual function has been linked to hyperglycemia, insulin resistance, chronic low-grade inflammation, endothelial dysfunction, neuropathy, and hormonal abnormalities. There are many different manifestations of female sexual dysfunction, such as insufficient sexual desire, diminished arousal, difficulty in eliciting orgasm, and pain during sexual engagement. Numerous studies have shown that the QoL of patients living with diabetes mellitus (DM) is lower than that of those without DM. SD in women with T2DM leads to deteriorated QoL. Treatment must be individualized based on the diagnosis and the sexual dysfunction as well as underlying medical, psychological, and interpersonal issues. The goal of modern medical care for patients living with diabetes is not to delay death but to improve their health and QoL. The present review article aimed to raise awareness about female sexual dysfunction in patients with T2DM and to provide an overview of its impact on QoL.

Keywords: female sexual dysfunction; type 2 diabetes mellitus; quality of life

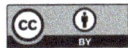

1. Introduction

Type 2 diabetes mellitus (T2DM) is a multisystemic disease with a high global burden. It is estimated that 500 million individuals are affected by the disease. T2DM has a bigger burden in developed regions (Europe, North America), with approximately equal gender distribution [1]. The pathophysiology of the disease can be explained as non-autoimmune progressive loss of insulin secretion against the background of insulin resistance and metabolic syndrome, which is stated in the American diabetes association guidelines [2]. Chronic complications of T2DM are numerous and they vary with respect to the duration of the disease and the adequate regulation of glycemia [3]. Complications impact the entire bodily system, encompassing the eyes, kidneys, nervous system, vascular system (involving both micro and macro changes), skin, bones, joints, and susceptibility to infection [4]. These complications have a profound influence on both quality of life (QoL) and overall life expectancy [1,3].

Sexual dysfunction (SD) in patients with T2DM is an often-neglected complication, despite the high impact on QoL [5]. SD is more common in men, with the primary symptom being erectile dysfunction, due to the complex intertwining of microvascular complications, autonomic neuropathy, low testosterone levels, and pelvic vascular disease [3,4]. Compared to male sexuality, the complexity of female sexuality is heavily influenced by psychological and societal variables. The interplay of neurologic, vascular, and hormonal systems is necessary for a normal female sexual response [6]. The prevalence and underlying mechanisms of female sexual dysfunction (FSD), as well as the associated risk factors in women with diabetes, are less clear than in men.

In the past 20 years, there has been a noticeable increase in interest in assessing and improving patients' QoL, particularly in chronic patients. QoL is one of the key indicators for promoting health and well-being in diabetic patients. Numerous studies have shown that the QoL of patients living with diabetes mellitus (DM) is lower than that of those without DM. Furthermore, a higher prevalence of sexual function disorder has been identified in the DM population, which may have a negative effect on QoL [7–11]. FSD frequently goes unrecognized and insufficiently addressed in women with T2DM. Healthcare providers may not routinely initiate discussions about sexual health, and patients may be reluctant to broach the subject, resulting in a deficiency of proper care [5].

This review article aims to heighten awareness regarding the issue of FSD in women with T2DM and to provide an overview of its impact on their QoL.

2. Type 2 Diabetes Mellitus and Chronic Complications

As mentioned earlier, T2DM is a multisystemic disease with a high global burden and an increasing prevalence worldwide. Chronic complications of the disease are a significant public health concern [1]. The rising prevalence of T2DM is associated with various risk factors, including obesity, sedentary lifestyles, unhealthy diets, genetic predisposition, and increasing life expectancy. T2DM has a substantial economic impact on healthcare systems and societies. The direct and indirect costs associated with diabetes management, including medications, hospitalizations, and lost productivity, are significant [1,3]. T2DM affects both men and women, but there are gender-specific aspects to its prevalence, risk factors, and impact on health. For example, postmenopausal women are at a higher risk compared to premenopausal women. This suggests that hormonal changes associated with menopause may play a role in the development of T2DM [1,4,7]. Furthermore, women who have experienced gestational diabetes during pregnancy are at an Increased risk of developing T2DM later in life. Women with polycystic ovary syndrome (PCOS), which is a common endocrine disorder among women, are at an increased risk of insulin resistance and T2DM [1,4,7].

T2DM can lead to a wide range of chronic complications, affecting various organ systems. These complications significantly increase the burden of the disease. T2DM can affect small blood vessels throughout the body, leading to microvascular complications such as retinopathy, nephropathy, and neuropathy [3,4]. T2DM is a major risk factor for cardiovascular diseases, including coronary artery disease, stroke, and peripheral vascular disease. It is a leading cause of heart attacks and strokes globally [1,3,4]. Diabetic nephropathy is a leading cause of end-stage renal disease (ESRD). It results from damage to the small blood vessels in the kidneys and can lead to kidney failure [3,4]. Diabetic neuropathy can affect both the peripheral and autonomic nervous systems. It can lead to sensory loss, pain, and autonomic dysfunction, affecting various body functions. Diabetic retinopathy is a leading cause of blindness in adults; it results from damage to the blood vessels in the retina and can lead to vision impairment or blindness if left untreated [3,4]. Diabetes-related foot problems, including neuropathy and peripheral vascular disease, can lead to foot ulcers and, in severe cases, lower limb amputations [3,4]. The chronic complications of T2DM can have a profound impact on the QoL for affected individuals. These complications often require ongoing medical care and lifestyle modifications and may lead to disability, reduced mobility, pain, and decreased life expectancy [1,3,4].

3. Definition and Prevalence

Female sexual dysfunction is defined as a persistent or recurring decrease in sexual desire, a persistent or recurring decrease in sexual arousal, dyspareunia, and difficulty or inability in achieving an orgasm [12]. The impairment of sexual function has been linked to hyperglycemia, insulin resistance, low-grade chronic inflammation, endothelial dysfunction, neuropathy, and hormonal abnormalities. These pathways can result in changes in genital blood flow, altered neuronal transmission, and decreased vaginal lubrication, all of which have an influence on sexual response [12,13]. A variety of psychosocial variables, in addition to diabetes-related physiological issues, contribute to sexual dysfunction in women with T2DM. Depression, anxiety, body image difficulties, marital problems, and medication-related adverse effects are among these variables. Furthermore, cultural and societal conventions around sexuality and diabetes may worsen emotions of guilt, stigma, and low self-esteem [12,13].

Female sexual disorders can affect women of reproductive age, which also include perimenopausal women. Menopausal and postmenopausal women are also affected by FSD. The biological and psychosocial components interact intricately to produce the human sexual response. Depending on the situation, these elements can differ between cultures, between people, and even within the same person [14].

FSD is divided into primary and secondary FSD. Primary disorders have symptoms that are not due to a medical or psychiatric condition or a substance, contrary to secondary disorders.

According to the older and more recent literature, the prevalence has not changed over the years. There are between 40–50% of women who suffer from some sexual disorders. In the United States, 12% of adult women (>18 year) report having a problem with their sexual function [15].

In women with T2DM, the prevalence of FSD is about 20–80%, compared to the general female population where it is about 40% [16]. However, a recent study by Derosa et al. showed that the prevalence of FSD is about 87% [17].

There are different tools to detect sexual dysfunction in females, so it is very important which questionnaire is performed; for example, the Arizona Sexual Experience Scale (ASEX) only measures the sexual function over the previous 7 days, whereas the Female Sexual Function Index (FSFI) measures sexual function over the previous 30 days, as well as which population is observed [12,18].

Quality of life is a complex concept defined by the World Health Organization (WHO) as an individual's perspective on life, including their values, aspirations, and standards [19]. It comprises various dimensions of a person's existence, encompassing the cognitive, physical, spiritual, emotional, and social aspects. In modern medical care for individuals living with diabetes, the ultimate objective is not merely to prolong life but to enhance their health and overall QoL [20]. SD in women with T2DM results in a decline in QoL, affecting critical physical, psychological, social, and spiritual aspects of their lives.

When we consider SD and its negative impact on the QoL, it primarily affects the social component and interpersonal relationships. It also affects women's self-confidence and self-awareness. At the same time, depending on the disorder, other domains of QoL are also affected, such as health, spiritual, and psychological components. To evaluate the effects of SD in women, the Sexual Quality of Life-Female (SQoL-F) questionnaire was developed using qualitative data. According to McHorney et al. [21], the 36-item Short-Form Health Survey (SF-36v2) is a widely used and extensively validated instrument designed for Health-Related Quality of Life (HRQoL) assessment. Thus, the most frequently used questionnaires for assessing the latter determinants are SF-36v2 and SqoL-F, both clinical- and science-wise [22,23].

4. Different Domains of Female Sexual Dysfunction

Different diagnostic and classification methods—the DSM (The Diagnostic and Statistical Manual of Mental Disorders) and ICD (International Classification of Diseases)—address organic sexual dysfunction. SDs are broadly classified in ICD-11 and DSM-V based on the stages of sexual activity, from arousal to orgasmic problems. In the following text, we will define four basic groups that belong to sexual disorders [24].

1. Desire disorders include a persistent absence of sex-related physical desire, a lack of sexual engagement, or sexual thoughts or fantasies that cause problems to patients and their partners. There are two main desire disorders: hypoactive sexual desire disorder (HSDD) and sexual aversion disorder (SAD). The questionnaire that can be used for this type of disorder is the Sexual Function Questionnaire (SFQ-V1) [25,26].
2. Arousal disorders are described as a lack of in sexual interest, interest in initiating sexual activity, pleasure, thoughts, and fantasies, including an absence of responsive desire and a lack of subjective arousal of a physical genital response to sexual stimulation: non-genital, genital, or both. The FSFI is the most used questionnaire for female arousal disorders [25,26].
3. Orgasm disorders: Female orgasmic dysfunction is characterized by an orgasm that despite normal levels of subjective arousal, is absent, rare, noticeably lower in intensity, or noticeably delayed in response to stimulation. They can be primary when women have never been able to have an orgasm, and secondary when women are no longer able to experience orgasms, despite once being able to. The female Orgasm Scale is the scale used for diagnosing orgasm disorder in the female population [25,27].
4. Involuntary contraction of the pelvic floor muscles when vaginal entry is attempted or completed, pain that is localized to the vestibule, at other vulvovaginal or pelvic locations, as well as fear or anxiety about penetration attempts are all symptoms of pain disorder. The Multidimensional Vaginal Penetration Disorder Questionnaire is used for determining sexual pain disorders [25,27].

5. The Effect of T2DM on Female Sexual Function

No definite mechanisms of T2DM on SD are yet known so, these are some of the proposed mechanisms (Figure 1).

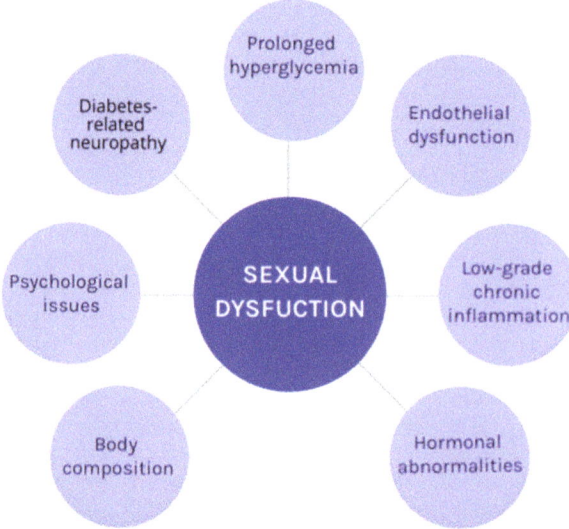

Figure 1. Proposed mechanisms of female sexual dysfunction in patients with type 2 diabetes mellitus.

The main mechanism is prolonged hyperglycemia, which causes cellular damage via a number of mechanisms, including advanced glycation end products (AGEs) and oxidative stress. This cellular damage has an impact on both the vascular and brain tissues involved in sexual response. Endothelial function can be impaired by AGEs, whereas oxidative stress can cause nerve damage, affecting the transmission of sexual inputs and feelings [5]. Hyperglycemia also decreases the hydration of mucous membranes in the vagina and increases the risk of infections, leading to problems with lubrication and dyspareunia [28]. Glycemic variability exacerbates vascular and neural damage, underscoring the importance of stable glycemic control to mitigate sexual dysfunction [29]. There are some studies that correlate better glycemic control with lower incidence of FSD and better outcomes [30].

It is well recognized that low-grade chronic inflammation has drawn attention as a possible mediator of endothelial dysfunction and cardiovascular disease in a number of metabolic diseases, including obesity, metabolic syndrome, and T2DM [3]. Endothelial activation, a pro-inflammatory state, and oxidative stress are caused by hyperglycemia, insulin resistance, hyperlipidemia, and poor dietary habits in both sexes. Through the combined mechanisms that cause damage to the genital area and hormonal abnormalities, diabetes may disrupt all these integrated systems, resulting in sexual dysfunctions [8].

Endothelial dysfunction, a hallmark of diabetes, influences the vascular health of the vaginal tissues. Reduced nitric oxide bioavailability and reduced endothelial signaling hinder normal blood vessel relaxation during sexual excitation, resulting in decreased vaginal blood flow and lubrication [12]. Diabetes-related neuropathy also affects the sensory and autonomic neurons responsible for sexual response, resulting in decreased sensitivity and altered genital reflexes [4,31]. A similar pathophysiological mechanism is observed in female patients with atherosclerosis and cardiovascular diseases. Atherosclerosis involves the buildup of arterial plaques, which can compromise blood flow to various organs, including the genital region, which ultimately leads to endothelial dysfunction and can lead to decreased genital sensitivity, arousal difficulties, and vaginal dryness [32,33]. It is therefore imperative is the early assessment of SD in patients to prevent complications of T2DM and atherosclerosis [16].

T2DM frequently causes hormonal abnormalities, which might contribute to SD. Insulin resistance and hyperinsulinemia affect the hypothalamic–pituitary–ovarian axis, altering sex hormone levels (mainly estrogen) and in the lower part progesterone and testosterone. Women with androgen excess and males with androgen insufficiency had the same cardiometabolic characteristics. The proper balance of estrogens and androgens is critical for maintaining energy metabolism, body composition, and sexual function. These changes can lead to diminished sexual desire, vaginal dryness, and poor genital responsiveness.

The psychosocial side of SD cannot be disregarded. The chronic stress associated with diabetes management, along with the psychological load of the illness, can lead to anxiety, despair, and poor body image. These psychological issues not only aggravate SD but also have an impact on hormone control, brain pathways, and general sexual well-being. The longer duration of T2DM aggravates those changes. Furthermore, SD can strain intimate relationships and disrupt partner communication. Feelings of frustration, guilt, and mutual dissatisfaction may arise, potentially leading to reduced relationship satisfaction. The resulting interpersonal challenges can ripple into other areas of life, affecting social support and overall relationship quality [9,10,13].

6. Sexual Disorders and Menopause

Following menopause, a woman's body and sexual urges may change due to the reduction of estrogen and testosterone levels in the bloodstream. Women who are menopausal or postmenopausal may realize that they are less amenable to being touched and that they are less quickly aroused, so decreased interest in sex may result from this [34].

Symptoms of menopause have a negative impact on QoL. Although women may also suffer changes in sexual function, temperament, and sleep, the most common menopause symptoms are vasomotor (such as hot flashes and night sweats) and genitourinary (such as vulvovaginal irritation and dryness, dyspareunia, and urine difficulties) [34].

A reduction in the blood supply to the vagina might also be brought on by reduced estrogens levels. That may have a negative impact on vaginal lubrication, making the vagina too dry for pleasurable intercourse. Accordingly, all of the mentioned sexual disorders can affect postmenopausal women: arousal, orgasmic desire, and pelvic pain during intercourse. It is essential to mention that disorders in menopausal women are secondary because of changes in hormonal levels in the bloodstream. Hormonal changes lead to changes in blood vessels and blood supply in internal and external gynecological organs [35].

Menopausal women have a substantially greater prevalence of FSD (63.9%) than women in of reproductive age (41.0%), with a 53.4% overall prevalence among women living with T2DM, as per Esposito et al.'s findings [36].

Women with T2DM can go into early menopause because of microvascular changes in the ovary. Therefore, ovary cells produce fewer hormones, such as estrogen and progesterone, than ovary cells in healthy women. They also have lower vascularization of the external genital organs, so they have vaginal dryness and lower clitoral stimulation [12]. Diabetes significantly alters the vaginal lamina propria vascular network, nitrergic signaling and androgen receptor expression, all of which have an impact on vaginal physiology. The higher risk of FSD development in women with diabetes may be caused by these changes [37].

7. Sexual Dysfunction as Per Gender

Although the distinctions between men's and women's sexuality, as well as their causes and etiologies, are not fully known, it is nevertheless feasible to make assumptions about these disparities. From various viewpoints, including biological, psychological, and biopsychosocial, one might examine sexuality. Although most researchers concur that both biological and sociocultural elements are important, they disagree over how much of an impact each has [28]. The impact of these various elements may differ for various sexual dysfunctions, for different life stages, and under various life circumstances [28].

8. Clinical Studies

The significance of DM in a woman's sexuality was largely ignored until 1970s. Kolodny started to publish on this topic in 1971 [38]. Then, in late nineties, Enzlin and others published a paper of SF in women with DM; since then, interest in the study of FSD in DM women has grown [39]. Results of several studies found the relationship between DM and FSD. A study, conducted by Shi et al., on FSD in Chinese women with T2DM found that diabetic women's overall scores for sexual function (SF) were considerably worse in the study group than in the control group [40]. According to a meta-analysis conducted by Pontiroli et al. that included 26 studies on 3168 diabetic women and 2823 controls, FSD is more common and is linked to a lower FSFI score in diabetic women than in controls [16].

Studying FSD in diabetic women has proven to be difficult because of the constant definitional changes, the exclusion of distress from studies of women's sexual dysfunction, and the high incidence of FSD in the general population as a result [4]. The lack of consistency in study designs among published clinical trials evaluating the impact of DM on women's sexuality makes it challenging to directly compare studies and draw conclusive findings.

FSD is relatively high in population without T2DM; therefore, study samples in patients with T2DM should be large to demonstrate this difference. Many studies have made no distinction between DM type 1 and type 2 [8]. The ability to account for the impact of the menopausal state and its treatment on sexuality is limited since authors usually combine pre- and postmenopausal women. The treatment of DM has changed in recent decades; consequently, women suffer less from SD. These variables may partially account for the variance in findings across research conducted at various times, and they raise the possibility that it may never be possible to compare studies conducted in different time periods.

In order to better understand the connection between DM and FSD, larger, more inclusive studies that include both women with DM and appropriate control groups are required. These studies should also use updated definitions of FSD.

Studies of women with diabetes have generally found weak or nonexistent correlations between sexual problems and age, duration of diabetes, body mass index (BMI), diabetic complications, medication, glycemic control, hormonal treatment, and menopausal status [31,39,41], in contrast to what has been found in studies on men with diabetes. However, in a study by Abu on 613 diabetic women and 524 healthy women, it was found that worse SF was significantly connected with longer diabetes duration, older age, higher BMI, the existence of cardiovascular problems, and the presence of diabetic sequelae [42]. Espasito found that metabolic syndrome and atherogenic dyslipidemia were independent predictors of FSD in 595 women with T2DM; nevertheless, depression and marital status were the two biggest independent predictors of FSD [36]. In contrast to male sexuality, female sexuality is much more complex and is greatly impacted by psychological and sociological factors, which was found in a review study conducted by Siddiqu et al.; it was discovered that psychological factors have a pathological predominance in sexual function issues in diabetic patients [43].

In the past two decades, there has been a rise in the attention given to QoL especially in chronic patients, which has prompted researchers to focus their efforts on identifying the elements that are most likely to improve it. In some studies, the association between SF and QoL in women at fertility age has been reported. Kiadaliri et al. observed that the QoL of diabetic patients was lower than that of their healthy peers in a systematic review study on diabetes in Iran [44]. Soltan et al., in their study, found no correlation between the SD and QoL in women with T2DM [45]. The current study set out to explore the relationship between sexual function and QoL in diabetic women seeking medical attention, taking into account the sparse and contentious existing studies in this area, as well as the cultural variations that have an impact on QoL and sexual function in various countries [8,9].

9. Interventions and Management

SD may indirectly impact diabetes management. Emotional distress and reduced self-esteem can lead to poor adherence to diabetes management strategies, including medication and lifestyle modifications. The resulting suboptimal glycemic control further reinforces the cycle of sexual dysfunction and decreased QoL [9]. Achieving and maintaining optimal glycemic control is essential for minimizing the impact of T2DM on sexual function. Effective management strategies should encompass lifestyle modifications, antidiabetic medications, insulin therapy, and continuous glucose monitoring to achieve stable glycemic control. By addressing hyperglycemia, one can positively impact vascular health, hormonal regulation, and neural pathways related to sexual function. Patient-centered care should prioritize open communication, individualized treatment plans, and sensitivity to the emotional impact of sexual dysfunction. Encouraging women to voice their concerns and providing tailored interventions can help mitigate the negative effects on QoL. These interventions are essential to improving the QoL of women with T2DM experiencing sexual dysfunction.

Other approaches have been integrated into the management of FSD, including medical and lifestyle modifications. Medical treatment options encompass hormone therapy, particularly in cases where hormonal imbalances contribute to FSD, leading to the prescription of hormone replacement therapy (HRT), such as estrogen [9–11]. Another option involves phosphodiesterase type 5 (PDE-5) inhibitors, commonly used to address arousal and orgasm difficulties in women due to their ability to enhance vaginal blood flow [9–11]. For women facing vaginal dryness or discomfort, topical estrogen treatments such as creams or rings can effectively improve vaginal health [9–11].

Lifestyle modifications are also crucial and include factors such as exercise, diet, stress reduction, smoking cessation, and moderating alcohol intake, all of which can have a positive impact on one's overall well-being and health. Over-the-counter products such as vaginal lubricants and moisturizers are available to alleviate vaginal dryness and discomfort.

Lastly, sexual aids such as vibrators or other similar devices can be beneficial for some women in enhancing sexual pleasure [9–11]. Psychological interventions play a vital role in the treatment of SD in women with T2DM. These interventions can address the emotional and psychological factors contributing to sexual dysfunction, help women cope with the challenges of T2DM, and improve their overall well-being. Interventions include cognitive-behavioral therapy, sex therapy, mindfulness and relaxation techniques, psychoeducation, and couple's counseling [9]. Addressing physical, psychological, relational, and societal dimensions is crucial. Multidisciplinary approaches involving healthcare providers, psychologists, sex therapists, and partners can provide comprehensive support. Foremost, raising awareness about the relationship between T2DM, sexual dysfunction, and QoL is vital [11].

10. Conclusions

SD in women with T2DM is a multidimensional issue that has significant effects on their general well-being and QoL. A thorough understanding of the underlying mechanisms, together with patient-centered therapies, is required in order to improve sexual well-being in this group. Healthcare practitioners may provide holistic treatment that enhances the overall quality of life for women with T2DM by addressing the complex interplay between diabetes, hormonal changes, physiological changes, psychological variables, and cultural effects. All of this will bring better compliance of the patients, better glycemic control, and above all, fewer complications of the disease. Most importantly, raising awareness about the relationship between T2DM, SD, and QoL in women is vital.

Raising awareness of SD, especially among female patients with T2DM, should lead to their seeking professional help and support as early as possible to improve their sexual well-being and overall QoL.

Author Contributions: Conceptualization, M.R., D.P., B.B., A.B. and M.M.; writing—original draft preparation, M.R., D.P. and B.B.; writing—review and editing, A.B., M.M., M.R., D.P. and B.B.; supervision, A.B. and M.M. All authors have read and agreed to the published version of the manuscript.

Funding: This research received no external funding.

Institutional Review Board Statement: Not applicable.

Informed Consent Statement: Not applicable.

Data Availability Statement: Not applicable.

Conflicts of Interest: The authors declare no conflict of interest.

References

1. Ong, K.L.; Stafford, L.K.; McLaughlin, S.A.; Boyko, E.J.; Vollset, S.E.; Smith, A.E.; Dalton, B.E.; Duprey, J.; Cruz, J.A.; Hagins, H.; et al. Global, regional, and national burden of diabetes from 1990 to 2021, with projections of prevalence to 2050: A systematic analysis for the Global Burden of Disease Study 2021. *Lancet* **2023**, *402*, 203–234. [CrossRef] [PubMed]
2. ElSayed, N.A.; Aleppo, G.; Aroda, V.R.; Bannuru, R.R.; Brown, F.M.; Bruemmer, D.; Collins, B.S.; Gaglia, J.L.; Hilliard, M.E.; Isaacs, D.; et al. 2 Classification and Diagnosis of Diabetes: Standards of Care in Diabetes—2023. *Diabetes Care* **2023**, *46*, S19–S40. [CrossRef] [PubMed]
3. ElSayed, N.A.; Aleppo, G.; Aroda, V.R.; Bannuru, R.R.; Brown, F.M.; Bruemmer, D.; Collins, B.S.; Gaglia, J.L.; Hilliard, M.E.; Isaacs, D.; et al. 3. Prevention or Delay of Type 2 Diabetes and Associated Comorbidities: Standards of Care in Diabetes—2023. *Diabetes Care* **2023**, *46*, S41–S48. [CrossRef] [PubMed]
4. Gardner, D.G.; Shoback, D. *Greenspan's Basic & Clinical Endocrinology*, 10th ed.; McGraw-Hill Education: New York, NY, USA, 2018.

5. Faselis, C.; Katsimardou, A.; Imprialos, K.; Deligkaris, P.; Kallistratos, M.; Dimitriadis, K. Microvascular Complications of Type 2 Diabetes Mellitus. *Curr. Vasc. Pharmacol.* **2019**, *18*, 117–124. [CrossRef] [PubMed]
6. Musicki, B.; Liu, T.; Lagoda, G.A.; Bivalacqua, T.J.; Strong, T.D.; Burnett, A.L. Endothelial Nitric Oxide Synthase Regulation in Female Genital Tract Structures. *J. Sex. Med.* **2009**, *6*, 247–253. [CrossRef]
7. Parnan, A.; Tafazoli, M.; Azmoude, E. Sexual Function and Quality of Life in Diabetic Women Referring to Health Care Centers in Mashhad. *J. Educ. Health Promot.* **2017**, *6*, 25. [CrossRef]
8. Maiorino, M.I.; Bellastella, G.; Esposito, K. Diabetes and Sexual Dysfunction: Current Perspectives. *Diabetes Metab. Syndr. Obes. Targets Ther.* **2014**, *7*, 95–105. [CrossRef]
9. Muniyappa, R.; Norton, M.; Dunn, M.E.; Banerji, M.A. Diabetes and Female Sexual Dysfunction: Moving beyond "Benign Neglect". *Curr. Diabetes Rep.* **2005**, *5*, 230–236. [CrossRef]
10. Kizilay, F.; Gali, H.E.; Serefoglu, E.C. Diabetes and Sexuality. *Sex. Med. Rev.* **2017**, *5*, 45–51. [CrossRef]
11. Vafaeimanesh, J.; Raei, M.; Hosseinzadeh, F.; Parham, M. Evaluation of Sexual Dysfunction in Women with Type 2 Diabetes. *Indian J. Endocrinol. Metab.* **2014**, *18*, 175–179. [CrossRef]
12. Rahmanian, E.; Salari, N.; Mohammadi, M.; Jalali, R. Evaluation of Sexual Dysfunction and Female Sexual Dysfunction Indicators in Women with Type 2 Diabetes: A Systematic Review and Meta-Analysis. *Diabetol. Metab. Syndr.* **2019**, *11*, 1–17. [CrossRef] [PubMed]
13. Kautzky-Willer, A.; Harreiter, J.; Pacini, G. Sex and Gender Differences in Risk, Pathophysiology and Complications of Type 2 Diabetes Mellitus. *Endocr. Rev.* **2016**, *37*, 278–316. [CrossRef] [PubMed]
14. Wright, J.J.; O'connor, K.M. Female Sexual Dysfunction. *Med. Clin. N. Am.* **2015**, *99*, 607–628. [CrossRef] [PubMed]
15. Shifren, J.L.; Monz, B.U.; Russo, P.A.; Segreti, A.; Johannes, C.B. Sexual Problems and Distress in United States Women: Prevalence and Correlates. *Obstet. Gynecol.* **2008**, *112*, 970–978. [CrossRef]
16. Pontiroli, A.E.; Cortelazzi, D.; Morabito, A. Female Sexual Dysfunction and Diabetes: A Systematic Review and Meta-Analysis. *J. Sex. Med.* **2013**, *10*, 1044–1051. [CrossRef]
17. Derosa, G.; Romano, D.; D'angelo, A.; Maffioli, P. Female Sexual Dysfunction in Subjects with Type 2 Diabetes Mellitus. *Sex. Disabil.* **2023**, *41*, 221–233. [CrossRef]
18. Elnazer, H.Y.; Baldwin, D.S. Structured Review of the Use of the Arizona Sexual Experiences Scale in Clinical Settings. *Hum. Psychopharmacol. Clin. Exp.* **2020**, *35*, e2730. [CrossRef]
19. Rummans, T.A.; Clark, M.M.; Sloan, J.A.; Frost, M.H.; Bostwick, J.M.; Atherton, P.J.; Johnson, M.E.; Gamble, G.; Richardson, J.; Brown, P.; et al. Impacting Quality of Life for Patients with Advanced Cancer with a Structured Multidis-Ciplinary Intervention: A Randomized Controlled Trial. *J. Clin. Oncol.* **2006**, *24*, 635–642. [CrossRef]
20. Kamalifard, M.; Sattarzadeh, N.; Babapour, J.; Gholami, S. Personal and Social Predictors of Sexual Function of Women with Type Two Diabetes in Sanandaj. *Crescent J. Med. Biol. Sci.* **2019**, *6*, 196–200.
21. McHorney, C.A.; Ware, J.E.J.; Raczek, A.E. The MOS 36-Item Short-Form Health Survey (SF-36): II. Psychometric and Clinical Tests of Validity. *Med. Care* **1993**, *31*, 247–263. [CrossRef]
22. Symonds, T.; Boolell, M.; Quirk, F. Development of a Questionnaire on Sexual Quality of Life in Women. *J. Sex Marital. Ther.* **2005**, *31*, 385–397. [CrossRef] [PubMed]
23. The Whoqol Group. World Health Organization Quality of Life Assessment (WHOQOL): Development and General Psychometric Properties. *Soc. Sci. Med.* **1998**, *46*, 1569–1585. [CrossRef] [PubMed]
24. Bhugra, D.; Colombini, G. Sexual Dysfunction: Classification and Assessment. *Adv. Psychiatr. Treat.* **2013**, *19*, 48–55. [CrossRef]
25. Montgomery, K.A. Sexual Desire Disorders. *Psychiatry (Edgmont)* **2008**, *5*, 50–55. [PubMed]
26. Rosen, R.; Brown, C.; Heiman, J.B.; Leiblum, S.; Meston, C.; Shabsigh, R.; Ferguson, D.; D'Agostino, R., Jr. The Female Sexual Function Index (FSFI): A Multidimensional Self-Report Instrument for the Assessment of Female Sexual Function. *J. Sex Marital Ther.* **2000**, *26*, 191–208. [CrossRef] [PubMed]
27. Grover, S.; Shouan, A. Assessment Scales for Sexual Disorders—A Review. *J. Psychosexual Health* **2020**, *2*, 121–138. [CrossRef]
28. Giraldi, A.; Kristensen, E. Sexual Dysfunction in Women with Diabetes Mellitus. *J. Sex Res.* **2010**, *47*, 199–211. [CrossRef]
29. Erol, B.; Tefekli, A.; Sanli, O.; Ziylan, O.; Armagan, A.; Kendirci, M.; Eryasar, D.; Kadioglu, A. Does Sexual Dysfunction Correlate with Deterioration of Somatic Sensory System in Diabetic Women? *Int. J. Impot. Res.* **2003**, *15*, 198–202. [CrossRef]
30. Veronelli, A.; Mauri, C.; Zecchini, B.; Peca, M.G.; Turri, O.; Valitutti, M.T.; Dall'Asta, C.; Pontiroli, A.E. Sexual Dysfunction Is Frequent in Premenopausal Women with Diabetes, Obesity, and Hypothyroidism, and Correlates with Markers of Increased Cardiovascular Risk. A Preliminary Report. *J. Sex. Med.* **2009**, *6*, 1561–1568. [CrossRef]
31. Erol, B.; Tefekli, A.; Ozbey, I.; Salman, F.; Dincag, N.; Kadioglu, A.; Tellaloglu, S. Sexual Dysfunction in Type II Diabetic Females: A Comparative Study. *J. Sex Marital. Ther.* **2002**, *28* (Suppl. S1), 55–62. [CrossRef]
32. Angulo, J.; Hannan, J.L. Cardiometabolic Diseases and Female Sexual Dysfunction: Animal Studies. *J. Sex. Med.* **2022**, *19*, 408–420. [CrossRef] [PubMed]
33. Allahdadi, K.J.; Tostes, R.C.; Webb, R.C. Female Sexual Dysfunction: Therapeutic Options and Experimental Challenges. *Cardiovasc. Hematol. Agents Med. Chem.* **2009**, *7*, 260–269. [CrossRef] [PubMed]
34. Chang, J.G.; Lewis, M.N.; Wertz, M.C. Managing Menopausal Symptoms: Common Questions and Answers. *American Family Physician* **2023**, *108*, 28–39. [PubMed]

35. Johnson, A.; Roberts, L.; Elkins, G. Complementary and Alternative Medicine for Menopause. *J. Evid.-Based Integr. Med.* **2019**, *24*, 2515690X19829380. [CrossRef]
36. Esposito, K.; Maiorino, M.I.; Bellastella, G.; Giugliano, F.; Romano, M.; Giugliano, D. Determinants of Female Sexual Dysfunction in Type 2 Diabetes. *Int. J. Impot. Res.* **2010**, *22*, 179–184. [CrossRef]
37. Baldassarre, M.; Alvisi, S.; Berra, M.; Martelli, V.; Farina, A.; Righi, A.; Meriggiola, M.C. Changes in Vaginal Physiology of Menopausal Women with Type 2 Diabetes. *J. Sex. Med.* **2015**, *12*, 1346–1355. [CrossRef]
38. Kolodny, R.C. Sexual Dysfunction in Diabetic Females. *Diabetes* **1971**, *20*, 557–559. [CrossRef]
39. Enzlin, P.; Mathieu, C.; Vanderschueren, D.; Demyttenaere, K. Diabetes Mellitus and Female Sexuality: A Review of 25 Years' Research. *Diabet. Med.* **1998**, *15*, 809–815. [CrossRef]
40. Shi, Y.F.; Shao, X.Y.; Lou, Q.Q.; Chen, Y.J.; Zhou, H.J.; Zou, J.Y. Study on Female Sexual Dysfunction in Type 2 Diabetic Chinese Women. *Biomed. Environ. Sci.* **2012**, *25*, 557–561. [CrossRef]
41. Olarinoye, J.; Olarinoye, A. Determinants of Sexual Function among Women with Type 2 Diabetes in a Nigerian Population. *J. Sex. Med.* **2008**, *5*, 878–886. [CrossRef]
42. Abu Ali, R.M.; Al Hajeri, R.M.; Khader, Y.S.; Shegem, N.S.; Ajlouni, K.M. Sexual Dysfunction in Jordanian Diabetic Women. *Diabetes Care* **2008**, *31*, 1580–1581. [CrossRef] [PubMed]
43. Siddiqui, M.A.; Ahmed, Z.; Ahmed Khan, A. Psychological Impact on Sexual Health among Diabetic Patients: A Review. *Int. J. Diabetes Res.* **2012**, *1*, 28–31. [CrossRef]
44. Kiadaliri, A.A.; Najafi, B.; Mirmalek-Sani, M. Quality of Life in People with Diabetes: A Systematic Review of Studies in Iran. *J. Diabetes Metab. Disord.* **2013**, *12*, 54. [CrossRef] [PubMed]
45. Soltan, A.Z.H.; Ranjbar, H.; Kohan, M. The relationship between sexual function of diabetic omen with quality of life. *J. Shahid Beheshtii Univ. Med. Sci.* **2013**, *23*, 32–39.

Disclaimer/Publisher's Note: The statements, opinions and data contained in all publications are solely those of the individual author(s) and contributor(s) and not of MDPI and/or the editor(s). MDPI and/or the editor(s) disclaim responsibility for any injury to people or property resulting from any ideas, methods, instructions or products referred to in the content.

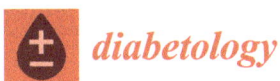

Review

Best Practices in the Use of Sodium–Glucose Cotransporter 2 Inhibitors in Diabetes and Chronic Kidney Disease for Primary Care

Jay H. Shubrook [1,*], Joshua J. Neumiller [2], Radica Z. Alicic [3,4], Tom Manley [5] and Katherine R. Tuttle [3,6]

1. Department of Clinical Sciences and Community Health, College of Osteopathic Medicine Touro, University of California, Vallejo, CA 94158, USA
2. Department of Pharmacotherapy, College of Pharmacy and Pharmaceutical Sciences, Washington State University, Spokane, WA 99202, USA; jneumiller@wsu.edu
3. Providence Medical Research Center, Providence Health Care, Spokane, WA 99204, USA; radica.alicic@providence.org (R.Z.A.); katherine.tuttle@providence.org (K.R.T.)
4. Department of Medicine, University of Washington School of Medicine, Spokane, WA 99202, USA
5. National Kidney Foundation, 6529 Linden Circle, Windsor, WI 53214, USA; tomm@kidney.org
6. Nephrology Division, Kidney Research Institute, and Institute of Translational Health Sciences, University of Washington School of Medicine, Seattle, WA 98195, USA
* Correspondence: jshubroo@touro.edu

Abstract: Diabetes is the leading cause of chronic kidney disease (CKD), with nearly half of all cases of kidney failure requiring kidney replacement therapy. While attention is often focused on the profound effects kidney failure has on the quality of life, the principal cause of complications and death among patients with diabetes and CKD is cardiovascular disease (CVD). These risks are often underappreciated by both healthcare professionals and patients. Sodium–glucose cotransporter 2 (SGLT-2) inhibitors were originally developed and approved as glucose-lowering agents for treating type 2 diabetes (T2D). However, agents within the SGLT-2 inhibitor class have since demonstrated robust benefits for CKD, atherosclerotic cardiovascular disease (ASCVD), and heart failure (HF) outcomes. Specifically, dedicated kidney disease and HF outcome trials have shown markedly reduced rates of kidney failure, CVD and HF events, and death among people (with and without diabetes) with CKD. SGLT-2 inhibitors will be used by primary care clinicians, nephrologists, and cardiologists across a range of cardiovascular and kidney conditions and diabetes. Knowledge and awareness of the benefits and key safety considerations, and risk mitigation strategies for these medications is imperative for clinicians to optimize the use of these life-saving therapies.

Keywords: diabetic kidney disease; type 2 diabetes; SGLT-2 inhibitors; albuminuria

1. Background and Introduction

Diabetes mellitus and chronic kidney disease (CKD), defined by sustained albuminuria (urine albumin-to-creatinine ratio (UACR) $\geq$ 30 mg/g), low estimated glomerular filtration rate (eGFR; <60 mL/min/1.73 m^2), or both for $\geq$90 days, commonly co-exist. Diabetic kidney disease, or CKD in diabetes without other known causes, occurs in about 30% of people with type 1 diabetes (T1D) and 40% of those with type 2 diabetes (T2D) [1]. CKD itself may be asymptomatic, but is associated with a high risk of morbidity and mortality. In the United States (US), over 37 million adults (~10.5% of the population) are estimated to live with diabetes [2]. Of these estimated 37 million adults living with diabetes, more than 90% have T2D [3]. Globally, 537 million people have diabetes, with a predicted growth in prevalence to nearly 783 million by 2045 [2,3]. As a global leading cause of CKD, diabetes accounts for nearly half of all cases of chronic kidney failure requiring kidney replacement therapy [4]. Despite the serious consequences of CKD, the low rate of awareness among clinicians and patients is troubling. Only half of patients at high risk for progression to kidney failure even know they have the condition [5].

When a person has diabetes and CKD, their risk for CVD events is equal to someone with established CVD, but it is even greater if the CKD is stage 3B or greater [6]. Therefore, patients with T2D and CKD are most likely to die due to cardiovascular (CV) events. Only about 10% of these patients will survive to progress to kidney failure requiring kidney replacement therapy [3,7,8]. The most common causes of death overall in patients with T2D and CKD are atherosclerotic cardiovascular disease (ASCVD) and heart failure (HF) [8]. A decline in the eGFR or the presence of albuminuria are additive risk factors for CVD events, CVD-related mortality, and all-cause mortality [9]. Even early stages of CKD in people with diabetes (stages 1–3) are associated with a dramatic increase in all-cause risk of death (3-fold) compared to people with diabetes and no CKD (hazard ratio (HR): 3.16; 95% confidence interval (CI): 3.0–3.4), and a loss of life expectancy of 16 years [10]. While the rates of most diabetes-related complications such as myocardial infarction, stroke, lower extremity amputation, and death have decreased in recent years, similar reductions have not been realized for cases of kidney failure [11].

Until recently, no class of glucose-lowering agents was considered a preferred treatment for patients with T2D and CKD. Rather, the recommended treatment approach focused on achieving individualized glycated hemoglobin A1c (HbA1c) targets, optimized blood pressure control, and the use of renin–angiotensin system (RAS) inhibitors, either an angiotensin-converting enzyme inhibitor (ACEi) or an angiotensin receptor blocker (ARB). The historical glucocentric approach focused on intensifying treatment in response to hyperglycemia in a reactive fashion, which means the treatment is always trying to catch up to the disease progression. Further complicating this approach, people with T2D and CKD have a more limited choice of glucose-lowering agents due to safety concerns (e.g., hypoglycemia, lactic acidosis with metformin) and other untoward effects (e.g., fluid retention with thiazolidinediones) in people with reduced kidney function. Treatment burden poses another significant barrier in patients with T2D and CKD. Many people with T2D and CKD require two to four medications to achieve and maintain individualized glycemic targets, another two to three medications to manage blood pressure, and yet another one to two to treat dyslipidemia [12]. Despite treatment with a large number of medications (which often also includes numerous medications to control or treat a host of other comorbidities), they still have large residual risk for death and CKD progression [13,14].

Fortunately for patients with T2D and CKD and the clinicians that care for them, major therapeutic advancements in recent years now offer additional options to mitigate kidney and CV risk. While initially developed and marketed as glucose-lowering therapies, SGLT-2 inhibitors are now recognized as "organ" (heart and kidney)-protective therapies. Consistent and robust evidence for markedly improved clinical outcomes have established SGLT-2 inhibitors as a first-line standard-of-care therapy for individuals with T2D and CKD [15].

2. Methods

The authors searched PubMed for all relevant clinical outcome trials in the last 10 years using the following keywords: type 2 diabetes AND: chronic kidney disease; nephropathy; albuminuria; cardiovascular outcome trials; heart failure outcomes; and renoprotection. The authors also utilized clinical practice guidelines published by the American Diabetes Association (ADA), the National Kidney Foundation (NKF), Kidney Disease: Improving Global Outcomes (KDIGO), and the American Society of Nephrology (ASN), American College of Physicians, American Academy of Family Physicians (endorsed ACP), BMJ, and Australia Diabetes.

3. Results

The authors reviewed the relevant literature and provided the following summative report. The goal was to highlight current evidence supporting the kidney and CV benefits of SGLT-2 inhibitors, highlight potential mechanisms of organ protection, and discuss important safety considerations when using SGLT-2 inhibitors for people with T2D and CKD. Finally, the authors discuss strategies to facilitate and encourage the use of SGLT-2 inhibitors to improve clinical outcomes in patients with T2D and CKD.

4. Discussion

SGLT-2 inhibitors work to lower glucose by preventing glucose and sodium reabsorption in the proximal tubule, leading to urinary glucose excretion and a reduction in blood glucose [16–18]. The US Food and Drug Administration (FDA) has approved five SGLT-2 inhibitors to date for the treatment of hyperglycemia in T2D: canagliflozin, dapagliflozin, empagliflozin, ertugliflozin, and bexagliflozin [19–23]. Based on findings from clinical trials, several agents within the class have received expanded indications (Table 1) [19–23]. Such expanded indications (depending on the agent) include reduced risks of: progression of CKD and kidney failure, heart failure hospitalization, major adverse ASCVD events, and CV or all-cause death.

Table 1. Labeled indications and dosing for currently available SGLT-2 inhibitors [19–23].

Agent	Canagliflozin	Dapagliflozin	Empagliflozin	Ertugliflozin	Bexagliflozin
Indication(s)	• Adjunct to diet and exercise to improve glycemic control in adults with T2D • To reduce the risk of MACE in adults with T2D and established CVD • To reduce the risk of ESKD, doubling of SCr, CV death, and hospitalization for HF in adults with T2D and diabetic nephropathy with albuminuria	• Adjunct to diet and exercise to improve glycemic control in adults with T2D • To reduce the risk of hospitalization for HF in adults with T2D and established CVD or multiple CV risk factors • To reduce the risk of CV death and hospitalization for HF in adults with HF with reduced ejection fraction (NYHA class II-IV) • To reduce risk of sustained eGFR decline, ESKD, CV death, and hospitalization for HF in adults with CKD at risk for progression	• Adjunct to diet and exercise to improve glycemic control in adults with T2D • To reduce the risk of CV death in adults with T2D and established CVD • To reduce risk of CV death and hospitalization for HF in adults with HF	Adjunct to diet and exercise to improve glycemic control in adults with T2D	Adjunct to diet and exercise to improve glycemic control in adults with T2D
Recommended dosing	• Initiate at 100 mg once daily • May increase to 300 mg once daily for additional glycemic control (if eGFR ≥60)	*Glycemic Control in T2D* • Initiate at 5 mg once daily • May increase to 10 mg once daily for additional glycemic control *All Other Indications* • Initiate at 10 mg once daily	• Initiate at 10 mg once daily • May increase to 25 mg once daily for additional glycemic control	• Initiate at 5 mg once daily • May increase to 15 mg once daily for additional glycemic control	• An amount of 20 mg once daily in the morning
Kidney dose adjustment *	• eGFR ≥ 60: No dosage adjustments required • eGFR 30 to <60: 100 mg once daily • eGFR < 30: Initiation not recommended; patients with albuminuria >300 mg/day may continue 100 mg once daily for organ protection • Contraindicated in dialysis	• eGFR < 25: Initiation not recommended; may continue 10 mg once daily to reduce the risk of eGFR decline, ESKD, CV death and HF hospitalization • Contraindicated in dialysis	• eGFR < 30: Use for glycemic control not recommended; data insufficient to provide dosing recommendations in patients with T2D and CVD • eGFR < 20: Data insufficient to provide dosing recommendation in HF • Contraindicated in dialysis	• eGFR < 45: Use not recommended • Contraindicated in dialysis	• eGFR < 30: Use not recommended • Contraindicated in dialysis

* eGFR values expressed in mL/min/1.73 m^2. **Abbreviations:** CV, cardiovascular; CVD, cardiovascular disease; eGFR, estimated glomerular filtration rate; ESKD, end-stage kidney disease; HF, heart failure; MACE, major adverse cardiovascular events; mg, milligrams; NYHA, New York Heart Association; SCr, serum creatinine; T2D, type 2 diabetes mellitus.

SGLT-2 inhibitors are efficacious glucose-lowering agents. In addition, SGLT-2 inhibition contributes to weight loss and modest reductions in systolic blood pressure [24]. While these risk factor benefits are well described, they do not fully account for the organ-protective effects of SGLT-2 inhibitors. This is evidenced by kidney and CV benefits observed in patients with CKD, where the glucose-lowering effects of SGLT-2 inhibitors are blunted (see Kidney outcome trials section below). Furthermore, several kidney and HF outcome trials have demonstrated benefits in people with CKD and in heart failure in the absence of T2D. SGLT-2 inhibitors can improve energy efficiency, reduce glomerular hyperfiltration and hypertension, increase erythropoietin and erythrocyte production, reduce oxidative stress, and reduce inflammation [25]. These proposed mechanisms may reduce fibrosis, podocyte and tubular damage, and mesangial matrix expansion in the kidney. In the heart, these effects are believed to reduce fibrosis, improve myocardial energetics, reduce myocardial remodeling, and improve left ventricular function [25]. While the mechanisms by which SGLT-2 inhibitors protect the heart and kidneys are still being explored, clinical trials support their central role in managing people with T2D, CKD, HF, and ASCVD (Figure 1) [26,27]. The following sections provide a succinct review of currently available clinical trial data (Table 2).

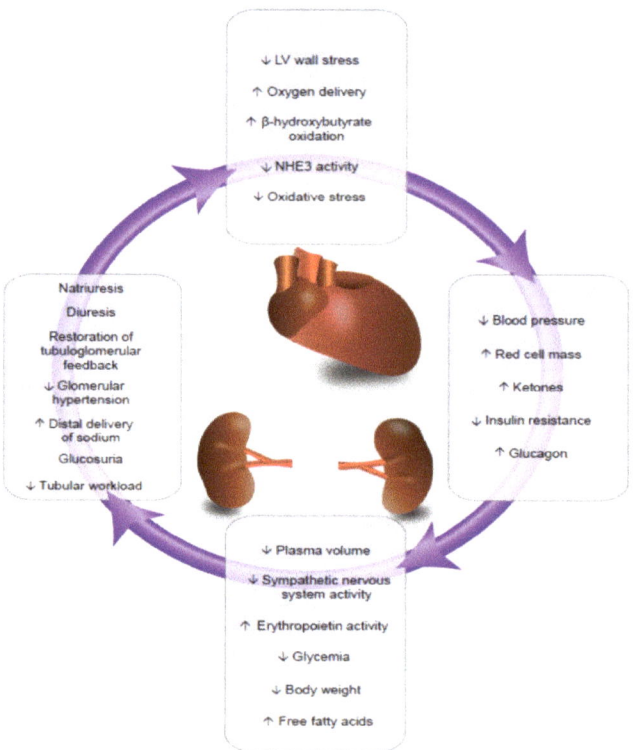

Figure 1. Mechanisms of kidney and heart protection by SGLT-2 inhibitors [26,27].

4.1. Cardiovascular Outcome Trials

Cardiovascular outcome trials (CVOTs) have been published for empagliflozin, canagliflozin, dapagliflozin, and ertugliflozin [28–31]. The EMPA-REG OUTCOME trial with empagliflozin was the first reported CVOT to demonstrate the safety of an SGLT-2 inhibitor, and the first to show the clear benefit of a particular glucose-lowering agent for protection against MACE in people with T2D and established ASCVD [32]. The trial's primary outcome was a composite of death from CV disease, non-fatal MI, and non-fatal stroke. The primary outcome occurred in 10.5% of patients in the intervention group compared to 12.1% of patients in the placebo group (HR: 0.86; 95% CI: 0.74–0.99; p = 0.04 for superiority) [32]. The CANVAS Program (canagliflozin) and DECLARE-TIMI 58 (dapagliflozin) trials reported benefits of treatment on CV outcomes [29,30] The VERTIS trial (ertugliflozin) demonstrated CV safety but failed to demonstrate superiority for its primary 3-point MACE outcome (HR: 0.97; 95% CI: 0.85–1.11) [31]. These CVOT findings have resulted in expanded ASCVD indications for canagliflozin and empagliflozin (Table 1). While findings of ASCVD benefits with agents from the SGLT-2 inhibitor class foundationally changed the treatment landscape for people with T2D, these landmark CVOTs also included key secondary outcomes of interest, including the progression of CKD and HF hospitalization.

4.2. Kidney Outcome Trials

In a follow-up to hypothesis-generating findings of kidney benefit in CVOTs, several dedicated kidney outcome trials have been completed with SGLT-2 inhibitors (Table 3) [33–35]. The first kidney outcome trial reported was the CREDENCE trial with canagliflozin [33]. CREDENCE demonstrated a superiority of canagliflozin treatment when added to standard-of-care background (optimized RAS inhibitor therapy) for the primary composite kidney outcome inclusive of end-stage kidney disease (ESKD), a doubling of serum creatinine, or CV or kidney disease death (HR: 0.70; 95% CI: 0.59–0.82) [33]. DAPA-CKD—which assessed the impact of dapagliflozin treatment on a composite kidney outcome (sustained decline in eGFR of $\geq$50%, progression to ESKD, or death from CV or kidney causes)—was tested in patients with CKD with or without diabetes [34]. When compared to placebo, dapagliflozin treatment reduced the relative risk for the composite kidney outcome by nearly 40% (HR: 0.61; 95% CI: 0.50–0.72). The number needed to treat was only 19 to prevent CKD progression or a kidney failure event over a median treatment period of 2.4 years [34]. CV-related death and hospitalization for HF was also substantially reduced, confirming both kidney and heart protection in patients regardless of diabetes status [34]. In further support of the findings from CREDENCE and DAPA-CKD, the Study of Heart and Kidney Protection with Empagliflozin (EMPA-KIDNEY) with empagliflozin likewise reported robust benefits of SGLT-2 inhibitor therapy in patients with CKD (inclusive of patients with and without diabetes) [35]. EMPA-KIDNEY reported benefits of treatment on a primary composite endpoint of CKD progression or CV death when compared to placebo (13.1% vs. 16.9%; HR: 0.72; 95% CI: 0.64–0.82) [35]. All three kidney disease outcome trials were stopped early because of the overwhelming efficacy showing clear, positive benefits for CKD with or without T2D. Therefore, CKD indications were added to the US labels for these agents (Table 1).

4.3. Heart Failure Outcome Trials

A series of dedicated HF outcome trials have solidified SGLT-2 inhibitors as a first-line standard-of-care treatment for HF, irrespective of diabetes status [36]. Four dedicated HF outcome trials have been completed with dapagliflozin and empagliflozin, demonstrating the benefits of these agents in both reduced-ejection-fraction HF (HFrEF) and HF with preserved ejection fraction (HFpEF), respectively [37–40]. The DAPA-HF trial reported a 26% risk of reduction in worsening HF or CV-related death (HR: 0.74; 95% CI: 0.65–0.85) in patients with HFrEF, and the DELIVER trial reported an 18% risk of reduction in worsening HF or CV death (HR: 0.82; 95% CI: 0.73–0.92), which are benefits largely driven by benefits on worsening HF [37,38]. Both trials enrolled participants with baseline HF with or without diabetes, with a benefit of dapagliflozin treatment observed irrespective of diabetes status in both trials. Similarly, both the Empagliflozin in Heart Failure (EMPEROR—Reduced) and (EMPEROR—Preserved) trials showed that treatment with empagliflozin decreased the risk of CV death or hospitalization for worsening HF in participants with HFrEF and HFpEF, respectively, regardless of the presence of diabetes [39,40]. Furthermore, the eGFR annual decline was significantly reduced in the empagliflozin groups [40]. A recently published meta-analysis of large HF outcome trials confirms the benefit of SGLT-2 inhibitor therapy to reduce the risk for CV death and HF hospitalization in a broad range of patients with HF [41]. As a result, dapagliflozin and empagliflozin are indicated for HF, irrespective of ejection fraction or diabetes (Table 1).

Table 2. Summary of SGLT-2 inhibitor outcome trials in people with T2D.

Agent *	CV MACE	CV Death	Kidney Disease Progression	HF Hospitalizations	Study/Refs.
canagliflozin	Reduced	No effect	Reduced (Primary Outcome)	Reduced (Secondary Outcome)	[29,33]
dapagliflozin	No effect	No effect	Reduced (Primary Outcome)	Reduced (Primary Outcome)	[30,34,37,38]
empagliflozin	Reduced	Reduced	Reduced (Primary Outcome)	Reduced (Primary Outcome)	[28,32,39,40]
ertugliflozin	No effect	No effect	No effect	Reduced (Secondary Outcome)	[31]

* Outcome data are not yet available for bexagliflozin. Abbreviations: CV, cardiovascular; HF, heart failure; MACE, major adverse cardiovascular events.

Table 3. Summary of key kidney outcome trials with sodium–glucose cotransporter 2 inhibitors [33–35].

Trial	CREDENCE (n = 4401)	DAPA-CKD (n = 4304)	EMPA-KIDNEY (n = 6609)
Treatment	Canagliflozin vs. Placebo	Dapagliflozin vs. Placebo	Empagliflozin vs. Placebo
Key Inclusion Criteria	• T2D • eGFR 30 to <90 mL/min/1.73 m^2 • UACR > 300 to 5000 mg/g • Treated with RAS inhibitor for ≥4 weeks prior to randomization	• eGFR 25 to 75 mL/min/1.73 m^2 • UACR of 200 to 5000 mg/g • Treated with RAS inhibitor for ≥ 4 weeks prior to screening	• eGFR 20 to <45 mL/min/1.73 m^2, regardless of UACR; OR eGFR ≥ 45 to <90 mL/min/1.73 m^2 with UACR ≥ 200 mg/g • Treated with background RAS inhibitor
Mean Participant Age (Years)	63	62	64
Baseline Diagnosis of T2D (%)	100	67	46
Median Follow-Up (Years)	2.6	2.4	2.0
Primary Composite Outcome			
HR (95% CI)	ESKD, doubling of SCr, or renal or CV death 0.70 (0.59–0.82)	≥50% decline in eGFR, ESKD, or renal or CV death 0.61 (0.51–0.72)	ESKD, sustained eGFR < 10 mL/min/1.73 m^2, sustained ≥40% decrease in eGFR, or renal or CV death 0.72 (0.64–0.82)

Abbreviations: A1C, glycated hemoglobin A1c; CI, confidence interval; CV, cardiovascular; eGFR, estimated glomerular filtration rate; ESKD, end-stage kidney disease; HF, heart failure; HR, hazard ratio; RAS, renin–angiotensin system; SCr, serum creatinine; T2D, type 2 diabetes mellitus; UACR, urinary albumin-to-creatinine ratio.

5. Guideline Recommendations for Use of SGLT-2 Inhibitors

In consideration of the glucose-lowering and organ-protective benefits of SGLT-2 inhibitors, this class of medication has taken a prominent position within current diabetes, CKD, and CVD guidelines (Table 4) [15,42–44]. A recently published consensus statement by the American Diabetes Association (ADA)/Kidney Disease: Improving Global Outcomes (KDIGO) on the management of CKD in diabetes recommends first-line treatment with an SGLT-2 inhibitor with proven kidney or CV benefits in patients with T2D,

CKD, and an eGFR ≥ 20 mL/min/1.73 m² [45]. Once initiated, SGLT-2 inhibitor therapy is recommended to be continued at lower eGFR levels until the patient progresses to dialysis [45].

Table 4. SGLT-2 inhibitor guideline recommendations for CKD and CVD in T2D [15,42–44].

Professional Group Recommendations	SGLT-2 Inhibitor Recommended: CKD	SGLT-2 Inhibitor Recommended: ASCVD	SGLT-2 Inhibitor Recommended: HF	SGLT-2 Inhibitor Recommendation Independent of Metformin
European Society of Cardiology/European Association for the Study of Diabetes Guidelines 2019	YES *	YES	YES	YES If patients drug-naïve for glucose-lowering agents
American Diabetes Association Standards of Care in Diabetes 2023	YES **	YES If GFR adequate based on drug approval label	YES If GFR adequate based on drug approval label	YES
Kidney Disease Improving Global Outcomes Diabetes and CKD Guideline 2022	YES **	YES If GFR adequate based on drug approval label	YES If GFR adequate based on drug approval label	YES
American Heart Association Scientific Statement on Cardiorenal Protection in Diabetes and CKD 2020	YES *** If GFR adequate based on drug approval label	YES If GFR adequate based on drug approval label	YES If GFR adequate based on drug approval label	No comment

* eGFR 30 to <90 mL/min/1.73 m². ** eGFR ≥ 20 mL/min/1.73 m². *** eGFR ≥ 30 or ≥45 mL/min/1.73 m² depending upon agent; for canagliflozin: eGFR 30–45 mL/min/1.73 m² and urine albumin-to-creatinine ratio > 300 mg/g.

6. SGLT-2 Inhibitors: Safety Considerations and Risk Mitigation Strategies

Important known side effects of SGLT-2 inhibitors include euglycemic ketoacidosis, genital mycotic infections, and volume depletion. For those patients with a prior history of these side effects, particularly if recent or recurrent, the balance of benefits and harms of SGLT-2 inhibitors should be discussed with these patients. This will allow for shared decision-making that can improve the safety and adherence to these therapies.

Euglycemic diabetic ketoacidosis (DKA) may occur in patients taking SGLT-2 inhibitors due to increased fatty acid oxidation and glucagon release along with decreased insulin secretion [46,47]. Patients with diabetes who are taking insulin are at the greatest risk of ketoacidosis. To reduce the DKA risk in T2D, it is important to maintain insulin treatment and pause SGLT-2 inhibitor treatment during periods of acute illness or other significant stressors. Patients with signs or symptoms of ketoacidosis, such as nausea, vomiting, and abdominal pain, should be instructed to discontinue SGLT-2 inhibitor therapy and seek immediate medical attention. Blood or urine ketone monitoring may be used for early detection of ketosis. One of the suggested strategies for addressing euglycemic ketoacidosis is the education of patients and clinicians on early recognition, and the implementation of the "STOP DKA" protocol (stop SGLT-2 inhibitor, test for ketones, maintain fluid and carbohydrate intake, use maintenance and supplemental insulin) [45]. Currently, SGLT-2 inhibitors are not indicated for use in the US, nor in the UK for people with T1D.

SGLT-2 inhibition is associated with an acute decline in eGFR of 3–5 mL/min/1.73 m² ("eGFR dip") due to a functional decline in glomerular hyperfiltration. Generally, kidney function stabilizes within several weeks. Importantly, this dip is not a reason for SGLT-2 inhibitor discontinuation [48–50], with patients experiencing relatively large initial dips in eGFR (e.g., >10%), deriving clinical kidney benefit [51]. SGLT-2 inhibitors can also cause volume depletion due to their diuretic effect. Stopping or reducing doses of other diuretics is generally not necessary upon SGLT-2 inhibitor initiation. Indeed, an analysis from the EMPA-REG OUTCOME trial found that SGLT-2 inhibitor therapy prevented CKD progression in patients with T2D and cardiovascular disease irrespective of common background medications that alter renal hemodynamics (e.g., RAS inhibitors, calcium channel blockers, diuretics) without increasing the risk for acute adverse kidney events [52]. However, the clinical monitoring of eGFR and electrolytes is prudent to inform dose titration and/or to adjustment of other antihypertensive or diuretic agents. Further, to minimize the risk of volume depletion, SGLT-2 inhibitor treatment should be paused during periods of acute illness or other stressors [53]. Genital mycotic infections occur more often in SGLT-2 inhibitor users (2–4% in men and 3–7% in women, versus <2% in non-users in both sexes) [54]. A recent report advised that the daily rinsing of the genital area after voiding and before bedtime significantly lessened the risk of genital mycotic infections (6/125 versus 51/125, $p = 0.015$) and also increased adherence to SGLT-2 inhibitor treatment over a three-year period [55]. A less common but severe side effect is Fournier's gangrene. This is a rare (1 in 10,000 patients), but serious, illness that was reported a post-market approval to the FDA [56]. It is unclear how much of this risk is attributable to SGLT-2 inhibitor treatment versus increased rates of skin infections in diabetes in general [55].

Primary Care Guidelines

While many specialists endorse and follow the above guidelines for care for people with diabetes, important primary care societies also provide recommendations for these patients. Some guidelines have not been updated recently enough to reflect the data. The American College of Physicians and the American Academy of Family Physicians follow the ACP guidelines published in 2017 [57]. The Diabetes Australia guidelines were published in 2020 and recognize the benefits of SGLT-2 inhibitors but list them as Class C [58]. The BMJ guidelines were published in 2021 and recommend the use of SGLT-2 inhibitors in people with CVD or renal disease or both [59]. It is important that these guidelines also be updated more regularly to reflect current trial patient outcomes.

7. Strategies and Considerations to Optimize Uptake of SGLT-2 Inhibitors

The clinical benefits of SGLT-2 inhibition can only be realized with appropriate use of these guideline-directed medical therapies. The first step is increasing awareness and identification of CKD. Health care professionals should screen for CKD by eGFR and albuminuria testing annually in persons with diabetes and others at high risk (e.g., hypertension, family history, CV disease). It is important to remember that an early response to kidney damage and glomerular injury is a hyperfiltration of the remaining functional glomeruli. Therefore, this makes low eGFR a late finding during CKD, and albuminuria may detect CKD earlier before eGFR decline. Once identified, the need for treatment may seem straightforward, but changing practice patterns is challenging. We have known about the benefits of ACEis and ARBs for over twenty years. However, even recently, the implementation of this standard-of-care for diabetes and CKD was striking low, in the range of 20 to 40% [27,60]. The need for a wider use of SGLT-2 inhibitors highlights the urgent need for better CKD screening and detection. Further, widespread patient education and engagement regarding the benefits of receiving RAS inhibitors and SGLT-2 inhibitors is needed. This can be accomplished via focused discussion and information dispersed in clinical settings, targeted information for high-risk groups, and public media platforms. In one such example, the NKF and CVS Kidney Care have partnered on a campaign to promote kidney health and screening for CKD [61]. Primary care clinicians are central in this effort to improve (CKD and CVD) outcomes for people with diabetes. Active early engagement from primary care and timely intervention can have a profound impact on the quality of life, morbidity, and mortality of these patients.

Key messages for providers to promote optimized use of SGLT-2 inhibitors in people with T2D and CKD:
1. Diabetes is the leading cause of CKD and kidney failure worldwide.
2. Few people at high risk of kidney failure know that they have CKD.
3. CVD is the leading cause of death in people with diabetes and CKD.
4. SGLT-2 inhibitors reduce the risks of progression to kidney failure, HF, ASCVD, and death.

8. Conclusions

Diabetes is the leading cause of CKD and kidney failure worldwide with high risks of ASCVD, HF, and death. CKD is a silent disease for most people and the targeted screening of eGFR and albuminuria is needed to identify it in people with diabetes and others at high risk (e.g., hypertension, family history, CV disease). SGLT-2 inhibitors improve glucose control and also significantly reduce CKD and CVD risks, irrespective of glycemic control or use of other glucose-lowering agents. SGLT-2 inhibitors will be also utilized in treatment beyond hyperglycemia. These agents are now first-line therapies for ASCVD, HF, and CKD, irrespective of diabetes status. Primary care clinicians should become comfortable with prescribing these agents along with cardiologists, nephrologists, and endocrinologists. A strong knowledge of benefits, side effects, and risk mitigation is needed to deliver optimal care of patients who take SGLT-2 inhibitors. Primary care providers have a responsibility to screen for CKD and implement SGLT-2 inhibitors in patients likely to benefit.

Author Contributions: Conceptualization: all authors; investigation: all authors; data curation: all authors; writing—original draft preparation: all authors; writing—review and editing: J.H.S., J.J.N. and R.Z.A.; input to final manuscript: all authors. All authors have read and agreed to the published version of the manuscript.

Funding: This research received no external funding.

Conflicts of Interest: J.H.S. reports he has been a consultant to Abbott, Bayer and Novo Nordisk. He has served on an advisory board for Abbott, Astra Zeneca, Bayer, Eli Lilly, Madrigal, Novo Nordisk, and Nevro. J.J.N. reports personal fees and other support from Bayer AG; personal fees from Sanofi; personal fees from Novo Nordisk; personal fees from Boehringer Ingelheim; personal fees from Eli Lilly; and personal fees from Dexcom outside of the submitted work. R.Z.A. reports consulting fees from Boehringer Ingelheim; and grant research funding support from the Centers for Disease Control and Prevention. T.M. is an employee of the National Kidney Foundation. K.R.T. is supported by NIH research grants R01MD014712, U2CDK114886, UL1TR002319, U54DK083912, U01DK100846, OT2HL161847, UM1AI109568 and a CDC contract 75D301-21-P-12254. She reports other support from Eli Lilly; personal fees and other support from Boehringer Ingelheim; personal fees and other support from AstraZeneca; grants, personal fees, and other support from Bayer AG; grants, personal fees, and other support from Novo Nordisk; grants and other support from Goldfinch Bio; other support from Gilead; and grants from Travere, all outside the submitted work.

References

1. National Kidney Foundation. KDOQI Clinical Practice Guideline for Diabetes and CKD: 2012 Update. *Am. J. Kidney Dis.* **2012**, *60*, 850–886. [CrossRef] [PubMed]
2. Center for Disease Control and Prevention. *2022 National Diabetes Statistics Report*; Center for Disease Control and Prevention: Atlanta, GA, USA, 2022.
3. International Diabetes Federation. *IDF Diabetes Atlas Tenth Edition*; International Diabetes Federation: Brussels, Belgium, 2021.
4. Hill, N.R.; Fatoba, S.T.; Oke, J.L.; Oke, J.L.; Hirst, J.A.; O'Callaghan, C.A.; Lasserson, D.S.; Hobbs, F.D.R. Global Prevalence of Chronic Kidney Disease—A Systematic Review and Meta-Analysis. *PLoS ONE* **2016**, *11*, e0158765. [CrossRef]
5. Chu, C.D.; McCulloch, C.E.; Banerjee, T.; Pavkov, M.E.; Burrows, N.R.; Gillespie, B.W.; Saran, R.; Shlipak, M.G.; Powe, N.R.; Tuot, D.S.; et al. CKD Awareness Among US Adults by Future Risk of Kidney Failure. *Am. J. Kidney Dis.* **2020**, *76*, 174–183. [CrossRef]
6. Tonelli, M.; Muntner, P.; Lloyd, A.; Manns, B.J.; Klarenbach, S.; Pannu, N.; James, M.T.; Hemmelgarn, B.R.; Alberta Kidney Disease Network. Risk of coronary events in people with chronic kidney disease compared with those with diabetes: A population-level cohort study. *Lancet* **2012**, *380*, 807–814. [CrossRef] [PubMed]
7. Packham, D.K.; Alves, T.P.; Dwyer, J.P.; Atkins, R.; de Zeeuw, D.; Cooper, M.; Shahinfar, S.; Lewis, J.B.; Heerspink, H.J.L. Relative incidence of ESRD versus cardiovascular mortality in proteinuric type 2 diabetes and nephropathy: Results from the DIAMETRIC

(Diabetes Mellitus Treatment for Renal Insufficiency Consortium) database. *Am. J. Kidney Dis.* **2012**, *59*, 75–83. [CrossRef] [PubMed]
8. Alicic, R.Z.; Rooney, M.T.; Tuttle, K.R. Diabetic Kidney Disease: Challenges, Progress, and Possibilities. *Clin. J. Am. Soc. Nephrol.* **2017**, *12*, 2032–2045. [CrossRef]
9. Fox, C.S.; Matsushita, K.; Woodward, M.; Bilo, H.J.G.; Chalmers, J.; Heerspink, H.J.L.; Lee, B.J.; Perkins, R.M.; Rossing, P.; Sairenchi, T.; et al. Associations of kidney disease measures with mortality and end-stage renal disease in individuals with and without diabetes: A meta-analysis. *Lancet* **2012**, *380*, 1662–1673. [CrossRef]
10. Wen, C.P.; Chang, C.H.; Tsai, M.K.; Lee, J.H.; Lu, P.J.; Tsai, S.P.; Wen, C.; Chen, C.H.; Kao, C.W.; Tsao, C.K.; et al. Diabetes with early kidney involvement may shorten life expectancy by 16 years. *Kidney Int.* **2017**, *92*, 388–396. [CrossRef]
11. Huang, E.S.; Brown, S.E.; Thakur, N.; Carlisle, L.; Foley, E.; Ewigman, B.; Meltzer, D.O. Racial/ethnic differences in concerns about current and future medications among patients with type 2 diabetes. *Diabetes Care* **2009**, *32*, 311–316. [CrossRef] [PubMed]
12. Harding, J.L.; Pavkov, M.E.; Magliano, D.J.; Shaw, J.E.; Gregg, E.W. Global trends in diabetes complications: A review of current evidence. *Diabetologia* **2019**, *62*, 3–16. [CrossRef]
13. Jafar, T.H.; Schmid, C.H.; Landa, M.; Giatras, I.; Toto, R.; Remuzzi, G.; Maschio, G.; Brenner, B.M.; Kamper, A.; Zucchelli, P.; et al. Angiotensin-converting enzyme inhibitors and progression of nondiabetic renal disease. A meta-analysis of patient-level data. *Ann. Intern. Med.* **2001**, *135*, 73–87. [CrossRef] [PubMed]
14. Lewis, E.J.; Hunsicker, L.G.; Clarke, W.R.; Berl, T.; Pohl, M.A.; Lewis, J.B.; Ritz, E.; Atkins, R.C.; Rohde, R.; Raz, I.; et al. Renoprotective effect of the angiotensin-receptor antagonist irbesartan in patients with nephropathy due to type 2 diabetes. *N. Engl. J. Med.* **2001**, *345*, 851–860. [CrossRef]
15. Kidney Disease: Improving Global Outcomes (KDIGO) Diabetes Work Group. KDIGO 2022 Clinical Practice Guideline for Diabetes Management in Chronic Kidney Disease. *Kidney Int.* **2022**, *102*, S1–S127. [CrossRef] [PubMed]
16. Cangoz, S.; Chang, Y.Y.; Chempakaseril, S.J.; Guduru, R.C.; Huynh, L.M.; John, J.S.; John, S.T.; Joseph, M.E.; Judge, R.; Kimmey, R.; et al. The kidney as a new target for antidiabetic drugs: SGLT2 inhibitors. *J. Clin. Pharm. Ther.* **2013**, *38*, 350–359. [CrossRef]
17. Gallo, L.A.; Wright, E.M.; Vallon, V. Probing SGLT2 as a therapeutic target for diabetes: Basic physiology and consequences. *Diab Vasc. Dis. Res.* **2015**, *12*, 78–89. [CrossRef] [PubMed]
18. Nauck, M.A. Update on developments with SGLT2 inhibitors in the management of type 2 diabetes. *Drug Des. Dev. Ther.* **2014**, *8*, 1335–1380. [CrossRef] [PubMed]
19. Canagliflozin (Invokana®) tablets. *Prescribing Information*; Janssen Pharmaceuticals, Inc.: Titusville, NJ, USA, 2022.
20. Dapagliflozin (Farxiga®) tablets. *Prescribing Information*; AstraZeneca Pharmaceuticals LP.: Wilmington, DE, USA, 2023.
21. Empagliflozin (Jardiance®) tablets. *Prescribing Information*; Boehringer Ingelheim Pharmaceuticals, Inc.: Ridgefield, CT, USA, 2022.
22. Ertugliflozin (SteglatroTM) tablets. *Prescribing Information*; Merck & Co., Inc.: Whitehouse Station, NJ, USA, 2022.
23. Bexagliflozin (BrenzavvyTM) tablets. *Prescribing Information*; TheracosBio, LLC.: Marlborough, MA, USA, 2023.
24. Neumiller, J.J.; Alicic, R.Z.; Tuttle, K.R. Therapeutic considerations for antihyperglycemic agents in diabetic kidney disease. *J. Am. Soc. Nephrol.* **2017**, *28*, 2263–2274. [CrossRef]
25. Alicic, R.Z.; Neumiller, J.J.; Galindo, R.J.; Tuttle, K.R. Use of glucose-lowering agents in diabetes and CKD. *Kidney Int. Rep.* **2022**, *7*, 2589–2607. [CrossRef]
26. Scheen, A.J. Cardiovascular effect of new oral glucose-lowering agents: DPP-4 and SGLT-2 inhibitors. *Circ. Res.* **2018**, *122*, 1439–1459. [CrossRef]
27. Tuttle, K.R.; Brosius, F.C.; Cavender, M.A.; Fioretto, P.; Fowler, K.J.; Heerspink, H.J.L.; Manley, T.; McGuire, D.K.; Molitch, M.E.; Mottl, A.K.; et al. SGLT2 inhibition for CKD and cardiovascular disease in type 2 diabetes: Report of a scientific workshop sponsored by the National Kidney Foundation. *Am. J. Kidney Dis.* **2021**, *77*, 94–109. [CrossRef]
28. Zinman, B.; Wanner, C.; Lachin, J.M.; Fitchett, D.; Bluhmki, E.; Hantel, S.; Mattheus, M.; Devins, T.; Johansen, O.E.; Woerle, H.J.; et al. Empagliflozin, cardiovascular outcomes, and mortality in type 2 diabetes. *N. Engl. J. Med.* **2015**, *373*, 2117–2128. [CrossRef] [PubMed]
29. Neal, B.; Perkovic, V.; Mahaffey, K.W.; de Zeeuw, D.; Fulcher, G.; Erondu, N.; Shaw, W.; Law, G.; Desai, M.; Matthews, D.R.; et al. Canagliflozin and Cardiovascular and Renal Events in Type 2 Diabetes. *N. Engl. J. Med.* **2017**, *377*, 644–657. [CrossRef]
30. Wiviott, S.D.; Raz, I.; Bonaca, M.P.; Mosenzon, O.; Kato, E.T.; Cahn, A.; Silverman, M.G.; Zelniker, T.A.; Kuder, J.F.; Murphy, S.A.; et al. Dapagliflozin and Cardiovascular Outcomes in Type 2 Diabetes. *N. Engl. J. Med.* **2019**, *380*, 347–357. [CrossRef]
31. Cannon, C.P.; Pratley, R.; Dagogo-Jack, S.; Mancuso, J.; Huyck, S.; Masiukiewicz, U.; Charbonnel, B.; Frederich, R.; Gallo, S.; Cosentino, F.; et al. Cardiovascular outcomes with ertugliflozin in type 2 diabetes. *N. Engl. J. Med.* **2020**, *383*, 1425–1435. [CrossRef] [PubMed]
32. Wanner, C.; Inzucchi, S.E.; Lachin, J.M.; Fitchett, D.; von Eynatten, M.; Mattheus, M.; Johansen, O.E.; Woerle, H.J.; Broedl, U.C.; Zinman, B.; et al. Empagliflozin and Progression of Kidney Disease in Type 2 Diabetes. *N. Engl. J. Med.* **2016**, *375*, 323–334. [CrossRef] [PubMed]
33. Perkovic, V.; Jardine, M.J.; Neal, B.; Bompoint, S.; Heerspink, H.J.L.; Charytan, D.M.; Edwards, R.; Agarwal, R.; Bakris, G.; Bull, S.; et al. Canagliflozin and Renal Outcomes in Type 2 Diabetes and Nephropathy. *N. Engl. J. Med.* **2019**, *380*, 2295–2306. [CrossRef]
34. Heerspink, H.J.L.; Stefansson, B.V.; Correa-Rotter, R.; Chertow, G.M.; Greene, T.; Hou, F.F.; Mann, J.F.E.; McMurray, J.J.V.; Lindberg, M.; Rossing, P.; et al. Dapagliflozin in Patients with Chronic Kidney Disease. *N. Engl. J. Med.* **2020**, *383*, 1436–1446. [CrossRef]

35. The EMPA-KIDNEY Collaborative Group. Empagliflozin in Patients with Chronic Kidney Disease. *N. Engl. J. Med.* **2023**, *388*, 117–127. [CrossRef]
36. Heidenreich, P.A.; Bozkurt, B.; Aguilar, D.; Allen, L.A.; Byun, J.J.; Colvin, M.M.; Deswal, A.; Drazner, M.H.; Dunlay, S.M.; Evers, L.R.; et al. 2022 ACC/AHA/HFSA guideline for the management of heart failure. *J. Card. Fail.* **2022**, *28*, e1–e167. [CrossRef]
37. McMurray, J.J.V.; Solomon, S.D.; Inzucchi, S.E.; Kober, L.; Kosiborod, M.N.; Martinez, F.A.; Ponikowski, P.; Sabatine, M.S.; Anand, I.S.; Belohlavek, J.; et al. Dapagliflozin in Patients with Heart Failure and Reduced Ejection Fraction. *N. Engl. J. Med.* **2019**, *381*, 1995–2008. [CrossRef]
38. Solomon, S.D.; McMurray, J.J.V.; Claggett, B.; de Boer, R.A.; DeMets, D.; Hernandez, A.F.; Inzucchi, S.E.; Kosiborod, M.N.; Lam, C.S.P.; Martinez, F.; et al. Dapagliflozin in heart failure with mildly reduced or preserved ejection fraction. *N. Engl. J. Med.* **2022**, *387*, 1089–1098. [CrossRef] [PubMed]
39. Anker, S.D.; Butler, J.; Filippatos, G.; Ferreira, J.P.; Bocchi, E.; Bohm, M.; Brunner-La Rocca, H.P.; Choi, D.J.; Chopra, V.; Chuquiure-Valenzuela, E.; et al. Empagliflozin in Heart Failure with a Preserved Ejection Fraction. *N. Engl. J. Med.* **2021**, *385*, 1451–1461. [CrossRef] [PubMed]
40. Packer, M.; Anker, S.D.; Butler, J.; Filippatos, G.; Pocock, S.J.; Carson, P.; Januzzi, J.; Verma, S.; Tsutsui, H.; Brueckmann, M.; et al. Cardiovascular and Renal Outcomes with Empagliflozin in Heart Failure. *N. Engl. J. Med.* **2020**, *383*, 1413–1424. [CrossRef] [PubMed]
41. Vaduganathan, M.; Docherty, K.F.; Claggett, B.L.; Jhund, P.S.; de Boer, R.A.; Hernandez, A.F.; Inzucchi, S.E.; Kosiborod, M.N.; Lam, C.S.P.; Martinez, F.; et al. SGLT-2 inhibitors in patients with heart failure: A comprehensive meta-analysis of five randomised controlled trials. *Lancet* **2022**, *400*, 757–767. [CrossRef] [PubMed]
42. Cosentino, F.; Grant, P.J.; Aboyans, V.; Bailey, C.J.; Ceriello, A.; Delgado, V.; Federici, M.; Filippatos, G.; Grobbee, D.E.; Hansen, T.B.; et al. 2019 ESC Guidelines on diabetes, pre-diabetes, and cardiovascular diseases developed in collaboration with the EASD. *Eur. Heart J.* **2020**, *41*, 255–323. [CrossRef]
43. ElSayed, N.A.; Aleppo, G.; Aroda, V.R.; Bannuru, R.R.; Brown, F.M.; Bruemmer, D.; Collins, B.S.; Hilliard, M.E.; Isaacs, D.; Johnson, E.L.; et al. American Diabetes Association. Standards of Care in Diabetes-2023. *Diabetes Care* **2023**, *46* (Suppl. 1), S1–S291. [CrossRef]
44. Rangaswami, J.; Bhalla, V.; de Boer, I.H.; Staruschenko, A.; Sharp, J.A.; Singh, R.R.; Lo, K.B.; Tuttle, K.; Vaduganathan, M.; Ventura, H.; et al. Cardiorenal Protection with the Newer Antidiabetic Agents in Patients with Diabetes and Chronic Kidney Disease: A Scientific Statement from the American Heart Association. *Circulation* **2020**, *142*, e265–e286. [CrossRef]
45. de Boer, I.H.; Khunti, K.; Sadusky, T.; Tuttle, K.R.; Neumiller, J.J.; Rhee, C.M.; Rosas, S.E.; Rossing, P.; Bakris, G. Diabetes management in chronic kidney disease: A consensus report by the American Diabetes Association (ADA) and Kidney Disease: Improving Global Outcomes (KDIGO). *Diabetes Care.* **2022**, *45*, 3075–3090. [CrossRef]
46. Fitchett, D. A safety update on sodium glucose co-transporter 2 inhibitors. *Diabetes Obes. Metab.* **2019**, *21* (Suppl. 2), 34–42. [CrossRef]
47. Rosenstock, J.; Ferrannini, E. Euglycemic Diabetic Ketoacidosis: A Predictable, Detectable, and Preventable Safety Concern With SGLT2 Inhibitors. *Diabetes Care* **2015**, *38*, 1638–1642. [CrossRef]
48. Nespoux, J.; Vallon, V. SGLT2 inhibition and kidney protection. *Clin. Sci.* **2018**, *132*, 1329–1339. [CrossRef] [PubMed]
49. Kraus, B.J.; Weir, M.R.; Bakris, G.L.; Mattheus, M.; Cherney, D.Z.I.; Sattar, N.; Heerspink, H.J.L.; Ritter, I.; von Eynatten, M.; Zinman, B.; et al. Characterization and implications of the initial estimated glomerular filtration rate 'dip' upon sodium-glucose cotransporter-2 inhibition with empagliflozin in the EMPA-REG OUTCOME trial. *Kidney Int.* **2021**, *99*, 750–762. [CrossRef]
50. Oshima, M.; Jardine, M.J.; Agarwal, R.; Bakris, G.; Cannon, C.P.; Charytan, D.M.; de Zeeuw, D.; Edwards, R.; Greene, T.; Levin, A.; et al. Insights from CREDENCE trial indicate an acute drop in estimated glomerular filtration rate during treatment with canagliflozin with implications for clinical practice. *Kidney Int.* **2021**, *99*, 999–1009. [CrossRef] [PubMed]
51. Williams, S.M.; Ahmed, S.H. Improving Compliance with SGLT2 Inhibitors by Reducing the Risk of Genital Mycotic Infections: The Outcomes of Personal Hygiene Advice. *Diabetes* **2019**, *68* (Suppl. 1), 1224-P. [CrossRef]
52. Dave, C.V.; Schneeweiss, S.; Patorno, E. Association of Sodium-Glucose Cotransporter 2 Inhibitor Treatment With Risk of Hospitalization for Fournier Gangrene Among Men. *JAMA Intern. Med.* **2019**, *179*, 1587–1590. [CrossRef] [PubMed]
53. Zoungas, S.; de Boer, I.H. SGLT2 Inhibitors in Diabetic Kidney Disease. *Clin. J. Am. Soc. Nephrol.* **2021**, *16*, 631–633. [CrossRef]
54. Harding, J.L.; Benoit, S.R.; Gregg, E.W.; Pavkov, M.E.; Perreault, L. Trends in Rates of Infections Requiring Hospitalization Among Adults With Versus Without Diabetes in the U.S., 2000-2015. *Diabetes Care* **2020**, *43*, 106–116. [CrossRef]
55. Murphy, D.P.; Drawz, P.E.; Foley, R.N. Trends in Angiotensin-Converting Enzyme Inhibitor and Angiotensin II Receptor Blocker Use among Those with Impaired Kidney Function in the United States. *J. Am. Soc. Nephrol.* **2019**, *30*, 1314–1321. [CrossRef]
56. Galbraith, L.E.; Ronksley, P.E.; Barnieh, L.J.; Kappel, J.; Manns, B.J.; Samuel, S.M.; Jun, M.; Weaver, R.; Valk, N.; Hemmelgarn, B.R. The See Kidney Disease Targeted Screening Program for CKD. *Clin. J. Am. Soc. Nephrol.* **2016**, *11*, 964–972. [CrossRef]
57. Qassem, A.; Barry, M.J.; Humphrey, L.L.; Forciea, M.A.; Clinical Guidelines Committee of the American College of Physicians; Fitterman, N.; Horwitch, C.; Kansagara, D.; McLean, R.M.; Wilt, T.J. Oral Pharmacologic Treatment of Type 2 Diabetes Mellitus: A Clinical Practice Guideline Update From the American College of Physicians. *Ann. Intern. Med.* **2017**, *21*, 279–290. [CrossRef]
58. Diabetes Australia: Best Practices Guidelines. Management of Type 2 Diabetes: A Handbook for General Practice. Available online: https://www.diabetesaustralia.com.au/health-professional-guidelines/ (accessed on 10 July 2023).

59. Li, S.; Vandvik, P.O.; Lytvyn, L.; Guyatt, G.H.; Palmer, S.C.; Rodriguez-Gutierrez, R.; Foroutan, F.; Agoritsas, T.; Siemieniuk, R.A.C.; Walsh, M. SGLT-2 inhibitors or GLP-1 receptor agonists for adults with type 2 diabetes: A clinical practice guideline. *BMJ* **2021**, *373*, n1091. [CrossRef] [PubMed]
60. Tuttle, K.R.; Alicic, R.Z.; Duru, O.K.; Jones, C.R.; Daratha, K.B.; Nicholas, S.B.; McPherson, S.M.; Neumiller, J.J.; Bell, D.S.; Mangione, C.M.; et al. Clinical Characteristics of and Risk Factors for Chronic Kidney Disease Among Adults and Children: An Analysis of the CURE-CKD Registry. *JAMA Netw. Open* **2019**, *2*, e1918169. [CrossRef] [PubMed]
61. National Kidney Foundation. *NKF and CVS Kidney Care Have Joined Forces to Promote Kidney Health*; National Kidney Foundation: New York, NY, USA, 2020.

Disclaimer/Publisher's Note: The statements, opinions and data contained in all publications are solely those of the individual author(s) and contributor(s) and not of MDPI and/or the editor(s). MDPI and/or the editor(s) disclaim responsibility for any injury to people or property resulting from any ideas, methods, instructions or products referred to in the content.

Commentary

Could Microbiome Be the Common Co-Denominator between Type 2 Diabetes and Pancreatic Cancer?

Marin Golčić [1,*] and Andrej Belančić [2,3,*]

[1] Department of Radiotherapy and Oncology, Clinical Hospital Centre Rijeka, Krešimirova 42, 51000 Rijeka, Croatia
[2] Department of Clinical Pharmacology, Clinical Hospital Centre Rijeka, Krešimirova 42, 51000 Rijeka, Croatia
[3] Department of Basic and Clinical Pharmacology with Toxicology, Faculty of Medicine, University of Rijeka, Braće Branchetta 20, 51000 Rijeka, Croatia
* Correspondence: marin.golcic@gmail.com (M.G.); a.belancic93@gmail.com (A.B.)

Abstract: Similar microorganisms, via similar mechanisms, play a role in the development of both pancreatic cancer (PC) and type 2 diabetes (T2D). Since the new onset of T2D is potentially one of the earliest signs of PC, it is highly plausible that a common denominator might be responsible for both, as the growth of the cancer will take a longer time to manifest compared to the insulin resistance. Although a variety of host-dependent factors and susceptibility play a role, and the mechanisms connecting the two diseases remain poorly understood, future well-designed trials should hypothesize whether a microbial intervention (modification and/or transplantation) results in a lower incidence and the better treatment of both diseases since the T2D–PC–gut microbiome interconnection seems scientifically logical.

Keywords: chronic inflammation; diabetes mellitus type 2; microbiome; pancreatic cancer; tool-like receptors

1. The Relationship between Diabetes and Pancreatic Cancer

Type 2 diabetes mellitus (T2DM) is a chronic metabolic condition characterized by hyperglycemia due to defective insulin secretion, the inability of insulin-sensitive tissues to respond appropriately to insulin, or both [1]. Due to its increasing incidence, T2DM is often referred to as the global epidemic of the 21st century, with an expected prevalence of 12.2% of the world's population by 2045 [2]. While the chronic health issues of T2DM are often associated with vascular complications, as almost 75% of all patients with coronary disease exhibit concomitant T2DM or abnormal glucose regulation [3], T2DM is also associated with a higher incidence of and worse overall survival (OS) for various cancers [4].

A particularly complex relationship exists between T2DM and pancreatic cancer (PC), the third leading cause of cancer death worldwide in men and women combined [5]. Despite the advances in modern oncology, the data from the largest phase III trials demonstrate a median OS of only 54 months after PC surgery [6] and 11.1 months after the diagnosis of metastatic PC [7]. Only several clinical trials with selected patient groups exhibited survival longer than 19 months in the metastatic setting [8]. Various factors influence the development of PC, including particular genetic drivers, family history, chronic pancreatitis, smoking, periodontal disease, drinking, and older age [9].

A long-standing T2DM is also associated with both the development of PC, with a relative risk of 2.1 (95% CI: 1.6–2.8) [10], and with a higher mortality of PC, particularly in patients with resectable cancer (HR: 1.37; 95% CI: 1.15–1.63) [11]. The relationship between the two diseases appears to be bidirectional as new-onset T2DM is associated with a significantly increased rate of PC diagnosis, particularly in the first 2 years after T2DM diagnosis (hazard ratio of 2.2 (95% CI 1.84–2.56)) [12]. On the other hand, removing both cancerous and normal pancreatic tissue after PC surgery improves related diabetic symptoms despite the loss of insulin-secreting tissue [13]. Hence, the data suggest that T2DM can both be part of the pathogenesis of PC and an early symptom and consequence of PC.

Despite the significant prevalence of both diseases, the data elucidating such a complex and bidirectional relationship are relatively scarce. For example, due to insulin resistance, an increase in insulin signaling pathways and insulin-like growth factor-1 (IGF-1) levels in T2DM can also lead to the proliferation and inhibition of apoptosis in PC, as IGF-1 receptors are usually highly expressed in PC cells [14,15]. Furthermore, T2DM is characterized by hyperglycemia, which does not increase neoplastic growth but can trigger oxidative stress, a factor in cancer pathogenesis. Additionally, several tumor-secreting products and metabolites such as amino acids, bile acids, and sphingolipids have been shown to be increased in PC after new-onset T2DM and could all play a role in PC development. On the other hand, developing paraneoplastic syndromes in PC can lead to insulin resistance [14].

Understanding the relationship between PC and T2DM in more detail could lead to earlier diagnosis and better treatment outcomes for both diseases. Hence, it is crucial to undertake research examining whether there is a common denominator linking both diseases. In this commentary, we suggest that the relationship between T2DM and PC should not only be looked at as bidirectional, as there is another significant factor at the root of both diseases, demonstrating a trilateral relationship—the microbiome.

2. The Importance of Microbiome in Pancreatic Cancer and Diabetes Mellitus

The microbiome comprises bacteria, archaea, viruses, and eukaryotes, which impact the metabolic and immune functions of the human body [16]. It has long been known that some of the bacteria in the gut microbiome can cause cancer, such as *Helicobacter pylori*, first identified in 1982 by Robin Warren and Barry Marshall [17], while other components of the microbiome have anti-tumoral potential [18]. While it was long thought that tumors are sterile, researchers have demonstrated the presence of microbiome in the tumoral milieu; this includes *H. pylori* DNA, which was found in 60% of patients with PC, suggesting that *H. pylori* may play a role in the occurrence of PC [19]. However, there are also data showing a higher prevalence of *H. pylori* infection in diabetic obese patients compared to nondiabetic patients (23.6% vs. 11.8%, $p < 0.001$) [20], suggesting that T2DM is a predisposing factor for the infection [21] and that the bacterium may be able to play its pathogenic role in the whole disease process [22].

A landmark study by Pushalkar et al. detected specific gut and tumor microbiomes in murine PC models, suggesting that a potential bacterial translocation can occur from the intestinal tract into the peritumoral setting [23]. Following these data, Riquelme et al. demonstrated that certain gut bacterial strains and a high microbial diversity can predict survival in patients with PC [24]. Furthermore, the same authors showed that fecal microbial transplantation (FMT), a method of impacting the whole host–microbiome ecosystem with capsules or an endoscopy from a particular donor, could modulate or shift the overall intratumoral bacterial composition. The performed FMT on the murine model demonstrated that applying the donor gut microbiota can influence tumor microbiota, tumor growth, and the level of CD8+ cells, the effects of which could be annulated by antibiotics. The effect shown was, in minor part, caused by direct translocation into the tumor through the bile duct and, more significantly, by altering the gut microbial landscape, shaping the immune response and promoting T-cell activation [24].

Dysbiosis of the gut microbiome also plays a significant role in T2DM. Qin et al. performed a metagenome-wide association study in 2012 in T2DM patients, demonstrating the presence of moderate intestinal dysbiosis characterized especially by a decrease in butyrate-producing bacteria and an increase in various opportunistic pathogens [25]. A Danish study evaluating the serum metabolome of insulin-resistant individuals found that dysbiosis of the human gut microbiome impacted the serum metabolome, systemic immunity, and contributed to insulin resistance [26]. FMT was also used in T2DM patients, showing that the colonization of the donor-derived microbiome via FMT could significantly improve insulin resistance, body mass index, and other clinical indicators in T2DM patients. FMT resulted in an improved microbial richness and Shannon diversity in the intervention group, while the relative abundance of Bacteroidetes was decreased and that of Firmicutes was increased after the intervention with FMT [27].

Oral microbes also play an important role in both PC and T2DM pathogenesis. Bacteria such as *Porphyromonas gingivalis* are important contributors to periodontal disease and may cause systemic inflammation. However, *P. gingivalis* is also shown to be associated with PC, as a comparison of PC patients and healthy controls demonstrated that higher levels of antibodies against a pathogenic strain of *P. gingivalis* were associated with a higher risk of developing PC (RR 2.14; 95% CI, 1.05–4.36) [28]. A similar effect was registered for *Fusobacterium nucleatum*, another periodontal pathogen [29]. On the contrary, higher levels of antibodies against commensal oral bacteria were associated with a 45% lower risk of PC when compared to those with lower levels of antibodies (RR 0.55; 95% CI, 0.36–0.83), suggesting that the presence of certain oral bacteria may actually decrease the risk of PC [28]. However, *P. gingivalis* is also shown to play an important role in the development of insulin resistance in mice fed with a high-fat diet through the synthesis of branched-chain amino acids [30]. Similarly, *F. nucleatum* levels are also positively correlated with fasting blood glucose and glycated hemoglobin, resulting in insulin resistance [31], demonstrating the role of oral pathogens in both T2DM and PC pathophysiology.

Along with gut bacteria, specific fungal microorganisms have also been associated with both diseases. Malassezia, the most prevalent fungal genus in PC, have been associated with the accelerated growth of PC via mannose-binding lectin, a soluble recognition molecule that binds to the terminal sugar residues present on the surface of microorganisms [32]. However, Malassezia is also implicated in T2DM, as the data show a high prevalence of Malassezia in patients with T2DM, with a lower number of yeasts in patients with adequate glycemic control [33].

3. Molecular Basis for the Trilateral Relationship

There are various mechanisms through which the microbiome can influence the development of both PC and T2DM. For example, microbial products such as short-chain fatty acids (SCFA) are dysregulated in PC, leading to the activation of the NF-kB signaling pathway, which can downregulate p53 expression and the level of inflammation [34]. A positive correlation between SCFA levels and a longer progression-free survival in patients with solid tumors were also registered in various studies [35]. On the other hand, Zhao et al. demonstrated that there is also a difference in the concentrations of microbiome and SCFA between healthy controls and T2DM patients. While the abundances of certain SCFA-producing bacteria were significantly increased in T2DM patients, the fecal SCFA concentrations were significantly decreased [36], which is important since SCFA butyrate can also provide a beneficial role in b-pancreatic cell function, as opposed to SCFA propionate which has a detrimental effect on diabetes risk [37].

The microbiota in diabetic patients also exhibited an increase in the oxidative stress response, potentially a direct link to the pro-inflammatory state of patients with T2DM. Moreover, diabetic subjects presented higher fasting and postprandial LPS concentrations than lean nondiabetic or obese subjects due to increased intestinal permeability [38]. Through a neuroendocrine pathway, increased gut permeability in T2DM patients can spread bacteria to other parts of the body. While the normal gut microbiota can dampen the nervous system's stress response, dysbiosis can result in an exaggerated hypothalamic–pituitary–adrenal reaction to stress, leading to an increased cortisol release and dysfunction of the gut barrier [38]. Parekh et al. previously showed that one of the earliest changes detectable in the evolution of T2DM is abnormalities in autonomic balance, which could be influenced by the gut microbiome [39].

Chronic inflammation and the response through toll-like receptors (TLRs) appear to be the central aspects linking T2DM, PC, and the microbiome. Chronic inflammation is associated with a phenotypic pro-inflammatory shift in bowel lamina propria immune cell populations [40] and the activation of different TLRs, which are innate immune sensors that recognize various stimuli and can both respond to invading pathogens and also regulate inflammatory responses and maintain epithelial barrier homeostasis.

TLRs have a complex relationship with carcinogenesis, as TLR4 and TLR7 are overexpressed by PC cells in both mice and humans, and exogenous TLR ligands can lead to accelerated pancreatic carcinogenesis in models of acute and chronic pancreatitis [41]. However, some TLR signaling pathways are tumor-suppressive, and due to a high degree of complexity and crosstalk with other signaling pathways, the overall outcome of TLR manipulation may not be easily predictable [42].

TLR4s are also expressed in insulin target tissues and are an important mediator of insulin resistance through activation by exogenous ligands, such as dietary fatty acids and enteric lipopolysaccharide, and endogenous ligands, such as free fatty acids, which are elevated in obese states. TLR4 activates the pro-inflammatory kinases that impair insulin signal transduction directly through the inhibitory phosphorylation of the insulin receptor substrate on serine residues and also leads to the increased transcription of pro-inflammatory genes, resulting in the elevation of cytokine, chemokine, reactive oxygen species, and eicosanoid levels; these promote further insulin desensitization within the target cell itself and in other cells via paracrine and systemic effects [43].

The microbiome exerts at least part of its physiological functions through TLRs, which means that the bacteria can potentially influence the pathogenesis of both PC and T2DM through the same pathways. Pulshakar et al. showed that various TLRs (3,4,7, and 9) are upregulated in PC, and that their activation accelerates oncogenesis via the induction of innate and adaptive immune suppression. Furthermore, the authors demonstrated that a distinct microbiome drives suppressive monocytic cellular differentiation in PC via selective TLR ligation leading to T-cell anergy, showing proof that the tumor-promoting effects of the PC microbiome are TLR dependent [23]. It was also shown that at least some of the carcinogenic effects of the oral bacterial strain *F. nucleatum* are due to TLR4 signaling, which can lead to the activation of the nuclear factor NFκB [44]. *F. nucleatum* has also been shown to induce cytokine release via the TLR2 signaling pathway, while also correlating with blood glucose and glycated hemoglobin levels [31]. Even fungal microorganisms such as Malassezia exert their function at least partially through TLRs, although specific data regarding T2DM and PC are lacking [45].

The relationship of the microbiome with both T2DM and type 1 diabetes is also regulated through the TLR signaling pathway [46], of which type 4 TLR-LPS signaling is particularly important and has been shown to mediate the metabolic benefits of caloric restriction [47]. It has also been shown that the deletion of TLR4 is associated with a higher abundance of Bacteroidetes and a lower abundance of Firmicutes in the large intestine, along with lower levels of circulating SCFA. Clinically, the deletion of TLR4 also results in insulin-resistance-related abnormalities in the energy metabolism [48].

4. Microbiome—The Common Denominator?

The data show that T2DM and PC patients exhibit signs of microbial dysbiosis. Although the relationship between T2DM and PC is likely bidirectional, complex, and multicausal, the finding that the new onset of T2DM is potentially one of the earliest signs of pancreatic cancer suggests that a common denominator might be responsible for both, as the growth of the cancer will take a longer time to manifest compared to the insulin resistance.

Evidence suggests that certain pathological bacterial strains can influence the development of both diseases, primarily through TLRs, which suggests that the microbiome might be a common denominator between the two diseases. Of course, various host-dependent factors and biological susceptibility play a role, and the mechanisms connecting the two diseases remain poorly understood. However, future trials could help to demonstrate the potential use of the microbiome as a screening tool, particularly for the oral microbiome, and could help to detect PC in earlier stages. Furthermore, we hypothesize that a microbial intervention might result in a lower incidence and better treatment of both diseases.

Author Contributions: M.G. and A.B. contributed equally to this work. All authors have read and agreed to the published version of the manuscript.

Funding: This research received no external funding.

Institutional Review Board Statement: Not applicable.

Informed Consent Statement: Not applicable.

Data Availability Statement: Data are contained within the article.

Conflicts of Interest: The authors declare no conflict of interest.

References

1. Galicia-Garcia, U.; Benito-Vicente, A.; Jebari, S.; Larrea-Sebal, A.; Siddiqi, H.; Uribe, K.B.; Ostolaza, H.; Martín, C. Pathophysiology of Type 2 Diabetes Mellitus. *Int. J. Mol. Sci.* **2020**, *21*, 6275. [CrossRef] [PubMed]
2. Sun, H.; Saeedi, P.; Karuranga, S.; Pinkepank, M.; Ogurtsova, K.; Duncan, B.B.; Stein, C.; Basit, A.; Chan, J.C.N.; Mbanya, J.C.; et al. IDF Diabetes Atlas: Global, regional and country-level diabetes prevalence estimates for 2021 and projections for 2045. *Diabetes Res. Clin. Pract.* **2022**, *183*, 109119. [CrossRef]
3. Standl, E.; Khunti, K.; Hansen, T.B.; Schnell, O. The global epidemics of diabetes in the 21st century: Current situation and perspectives. *Eur. J. Prev. Cardiol.* **2019**, *26*, 7–14. [CrossRef] [PubMed]
4. Abudawood, M. Diabetes and cancer: A comprehensive review. *J. Res. Med. Sci.* **2019**, *24*, 94. [CrossRef] [PubMed]
5. Siegel, R.L.; Miller, K.D.; Wagle, N.S.; Jemal, A. Cancer statistics, 2023. *CA Cancer J. Clin.* **2023**, *73*, 17–48. [CrossRef]
6. Conroy, T.; Hammel, P.; Hebbar, M.; Ben Abdelghani, M.; Wei, A.C.; Raoul, J.L.; Choné, L.; Francois, E.; Artru, P.; Biagi, J.J.; et al. FOLFIRINOX or Gemcitabine as Adjuvant Therapy for Pancreatic Cancer. *N. Engl. J. Med.* **2018**, *379*, 2395–2406. [CrossRef]
7. Conroy, T.; Desseigne, F.; Ychou, M.; Bouché, O.; Guimbaud, R.; Bécouarn, Y.; Adenis, A.; Raoul, J.L.; Gourgou-Bourgade, S.; de la Fouchardière, C.; et al. FOLFIRINOX versus gemcitabine for metastatic pancreatic cancer. *N. Engl. J. Med.* **2011**, *364*, 1817–1825. [CrossRef]
8. Kindler, H.L.; Hammel, P.; Reni, M.; Van Cutsem, E.; Macarulla, T.; Hall, M.J.; Park, J.O.; Hochhauser, D.; Arnold, D.; Oh, D.Y.; et al. Overall Survival Results from the POLO Trial: A Phase III Study of Active Maintenance Olaparib Versus Placebo for Germline BRCA-Mutated Metastatic Pancreatic Cancer. *J. Clin. Oncol.* **2022**, *40*, 3929–3939. [CrossRef]
9. Capasso, M.; Franceschi, M.; Rodriguez-Castro, K.I.; Crafa, P.; Cambiè, G.; Miraglia, C.; Barchi, A.; Nouvenne, A.; Leandro, G.; Meschi, T.; et al. Epidemiology and risk factors of pancreatic cancer. *Acta Biomed.* **2018**, *89*, 141–146. [CrossRef]
10. Everhart, J.; Wright, D. Diabetes mellitus as a risk factor for pancreatic cancer. A meta-analysis. *JAMA* **1995**, *273*, 1605–1609. [CrossRef]
11. Mao, Y.; Tao, M.; Jia, X.; Xu, H.; Chen, K.; Tang, H.; Li, D. Effect of Diabetes Mellitus on Survival in Patients with Pancreatic Cancer: A Systematic Review and Meta-analysis. *Sci. Rep.* **2015**, *5*, 17102. [CrossRef] [PubMed]
12. Gupta, S.; Vittinghoff, E.; Bertenthal, D.; Corley, D.; Shen, H.; Walter, L.C.; McQuaid, K. New-onset diabetes and pancreatic cancer. *Clin. Gastroenterol. Hepatol.* **2006**, *4*, 1366–1372; quiz 1301. [CrossRef] [PubMed]
13. Khadka, R.; Tian, W.; Hao, X.; Koirala, R. Risk factor, early diagnosis and overall survival on outcome of association between pancreatic cancer and diabetes mellitus: Changes and advances, a review. *Int. J. Surg.* **2018**, *52*, 342–346. [CrossRef] [PubMed]
14. Kaleru, T.; Vankeshwaram, V.K.; Maheshwary, A.; Mohite, D.; Khan, S. Diabetes Mellitus in the Middle-Aged and Elderly Population (>45 Years) and Its Association with Pancreatic Cancer: An Updated Review. *Cureus* **2020**, *12*, e8884. [CrossRef]
15. Gong, J.; Robbins, L.A.; Lugea, A.; Waldron, R.T.; Jeon, C.Y.; Pandol, S.J. Diabetes, pancreatic cancer, and metformin therapy. *Front. Physiol.* **2014**, *5*, 426. [CrossRef] [PubMed]
16. Ogunrinola, G.A.; Oyewale, J.O.; Oshamika, O.O.; Olasehinde, G.I. The Human Microbiome and Its Impacts on Health. *Int. J. Microbiol.* **2020**, *2020*, 8045646. [CrossRef] [PubMed]
17. Marshall, B.J.; Warren, J.R. Unidentified curved bacilli in the stomach of patients with gastritis and peptic ulceration. *Lancet* **1984**, *1*, 1311–1315. [CrossRef]
18. Vivarelli, S.; Salemi, R.; Candido, S.; Falzone, L.; Santagati, M.; Stefani, S.; Torino, F.; Banna, G.L.; Tonini, G.; Libra, M. Gut Microbiota and Cancer: From Pathogenesis to Therapy. *Cancers* **2019**, *11*, 38. [CrossRef]
19. Nilsson, H.O.; Stenram, U.; Ihse, I.; Wadstrom, T. Helicobacter species ribosomal DNA in the pancreas, stomach and duodenum of pancreatic cancer patients. *World J. Gastroenterol.* **2006**, *12*, 3038–3043. [CrossRef]
20. Bener, A.; Micallef, R.; Afifi, M.; Derbala, M.; Al-Mulla, H.M.; Usmani, M.A. Association between type 2 diabetes mellitus and *Helicobacter pylori* infection. *Turk. J. Gastroenterol.* **2007**, *18*, 225–229.
21. Sahoo, O.S.; Mitra, R.; Bhattacharjee, A.; Kar, S.; Mukherjee, O. Is Diabetes Mellitus a Predisposing Factor for *Helicobacter pylori* Infections. *Curr. Diab Rep.* **2023**, *23*, 195–205. [CrossRef] [PubMed]
22. Wang, F.; Liu, J.; Lv, Z. Association of *Helicobacter pylori* infection with diabetes mellitus and diabetic nephropathy: A meta-analysis of 39 studies involving more than 20,000 participants. *Scand. J. Infect. Dis.* **2013**, *45*, 930–938. [CrossRef] [PubMed]

23. Pushalkar, S.; Hundeyin, M.; Daley, D.; Zambirinis, C.P.; Kurz, E.; Mishra, A.; Mohan, N.; Aykut, B.; Usyk, M.; Torres, L.E.; et al. The Pancreatic Cancer Microbiome Promotes Oncogenesis by Induction of Innate and Adaptive Immune Suppression. *Cancer Discov.* **2018**, *8*, 403–416. [CrossRef]
24. Riquelme, E.; Zhang, Y.; Zhang, L.; Montiel, M.; Zoltan, M.; Dong, W.; Quesada, P.; Sahin, I.; Chandra, V.; San Lucas, A.; et al. Tumor Microbiome Diversity and Composition Influence Pancreatic Cancer Outcomes. *Cell* **2019**, *178*, 795–806.e12. [CrossRef] [PubMed]
25. Qin, J.; Li, Y.; Cai, Z.; Li, S.; Zhu, J.; Zhang, F.; Liang, S.; Zhang, W.; Guan, Y.; Shen, D.; et al. A metagenome-wide association study of gut microbiota in type 2 diabetes. *Nature* **2012**, *490*, 55–60. [CrossRef] [PubMed]
26. Pedersen, H.K.; Gudmundsdottir, V.; Nielsen, H.B.; Hyotylainen, T.; Nielsen, T.; Jensen, B.A.; Forslund, K.; Hildebrand, F.; Prifti, E.; Falony, G.; et al. Human gut microbes impact host serum metabolome and insulin sensitivity. *Nature* **2016**, *535*, 376–381. [CrossRef] [PubMed]
27. Wu, Z.; Zhang, B.; Chen, F.; Xia, R.; Zhu, D.; Chen, B.; Lin, A.; Zheng, C.; Hou, D.; Li, X.; et al. Fecal microbiota transplantation reverses insulin resistance in type 2 diabetes: A randomized, controlled, prospective study. *Front. Cell Infect. Microbiol.* **2022**, *12*, 1089991. [CrossRef]
28. Michaud, D.S.; Izard, J.; Wilhelm-Benartzi, C.S.; You, D.H.; Grote, V.A.; Tjønneland, A.; Dahm, C.C.; Overvad, K.; Jenab, M.; Fedirko, V.; et al. Plasma antibodies to oral bacteria and risk of pancreatic cancer in a large European prospective cohort study. *Gut* **2013**, *62*, 1764–1770. [CrossRef]
29. Mitsuhashi, K.; Nosho, K.; Sukawa, Y.; Matsunaga, Y.; Ito, M.; Kurihara, H.; Kanno, S.; Igarashi, H.; Naito, T.; Adachi, Y.; et al. Association of Fusobacterium species in pancreatic cancer tissues with molecular features and prognosis. *Oncotarget* **2015**, *6*, 7209–7220. [CrossRef]
30. Tian, J.; Liu, C.; Zheng, X.; Jia, X.; Peng, X.; Yang, R.; Zhou, X.; Xu, X. Porphyromonas gingivalis Induces Insulin Resistance by Increasing BCAA Levels in Mice. *J. Dent. Res.* **2020**, *99*, 839–846. [CrossRef]
31. Chang, Y.R.; Cheng, W.C.; Hsiao, Y.C.; Su, G.W.; Lin, S.J.; Wei, Y.S.; Chou, H.C.; Lin, H.P.; Lin, G.Y.; Chan, H.L. Links between oral microbiome and insulin resistance: Involvement of MAP kinase signaling pathway. *Biochimie* **2023**, *214 Pt. B*, 134–144. [CrossRef]
32. Wang, H.; Capula, M.; Krom, B.P.; Yee, D.; Giovannetti, E.; Deng, D. Of fungi and men: Role of fungi in pancreatic cancer carcinogenesis. *Ann. Transl. Med.* **2020**, *8*, 1257. [CrossRef] [PubMed]
33. Bello-Hernández, Y.; García-Valdés, L.; Cruz, S.; Pérez, D.; Vega, D.; Torres, E.; Fernández, R.; Arenas, R. Prevalencia de *Malassezia* spp en pacientes con diabetes mellitus tipo 2 de acuerdo con el control glucémico. *Med. Int. Méx* **2017**, *33*, 612–617. [CrossRef]
34. Temel, H.Y.; Kaymak, Ö.; Kaplan, S.; Bahcivanci, B.; Gkoutos, G.V.; Acharjee, A. Role of microbiota and microbiota-derived short-chain fatty acids in PDAC. *Cancer Med.* **2023**, *12*, 5661–5675. [CrossRef] [PubMed]
35. Nomura, M.; Nagatomo, R.; Doi, K.; Shimizu, J.; Baba, K.; Saito, T.; Matsumoto, S.; Inoue, K.; Muto, M. Association of Short-Chain Fatty Acids in the Gut Microbiome with Clinical Response to Treatment with Nivolumab or Pembrolizumab in Patients With Solid Cancer Tumors. *JAMA Netw. Open* **2020**, *3*, e202895. [CrossRef] [PubMed]
36. Zhao, L.; Lou, H.; Peng, Y.; Chen, S.; Zhang, Y.; Li, X. Comprehensive relationships between gut microbiome and faecal metabolome in individuals with type 2 diabetes and its complications. *Endocrine* **2019**, *66*, 526–537. [CrossRef] [PubMed]
37. Liu, J.L.; Segovia, I.; Yuan, X.L.; Gao, Z.H. Controversial Roles of Gut Microbiota-Derived Short-Chain Fatty Acids (SCFAs) on Pancreatic β-Cell Growth and Insulin Secretion. *Int. J. Mol. Sci.* **2020**, *21*, 910. [CrossRef]
38. Zhang, S.; Cai, Y.; Meng, C.; Ding, X.; Huang, Y.; Luo, X.; Cao, Y.; Gao, F.; Zou, M. The role of the microbiome in diabetes mellitus. *Diabetes Res. Clin. Pract.* **2021**, *172*, 108645. [CrossRef]
39. Parekh, P.J.; Nayi, V.R.; Johnson, D.A.; Vinik, A.I. The Role of Gut Microflora and the Cholinergic Anti-inflammatory Neuroendocrine System in Diabetes Mellitus. *Front. Endocrinol.* **2016**, *7*, 55. [CrossRef]
40. Luck, H.; Tsai, S.; Chung, J.; Clemente-Casares, X.; Ghazarian, M.; Revelo, X.S.; Lei, H.; Luk, C.T.; Shi, S.Y.; Surendra, A.; et al. Regulation of obesity-related insulin resistance with gut anti-inflammatory agents. *Cell Metab.* **2015**, *21*, 527–542. [CrossRef]
41. Li, T.T.; Ogino, S.; Qian, Z.R. Toll-like receptor signaling in colorectal cancer: Carcinogenesis to cancer therapy. *World J. Gastroenterol.* **2014**, *20*, 17699–17708. [CrossRef] [PubMed]
42. Zambirinis, C.P.; Miller, G. Signaling via MYD88 in the pancreatic tumor microenvironment: A double-edged sword. *Oncoimmunology* **2013**, *2*, e22567. [CrossRef] [PubMed]
43. Kim, J.J.; Sears, D.D. TLR4 and Insulin Resistance. *Gastroenterol. Res. Pract.* **2010**, *2010*, 212563. [CrossRef] [PubMed]
44. Yang, Y.; Weng, W.; Peng, J.; Hong, L.; Yang, L.; Toiyama, Y.; Gao, R.; Liu, M.; Yin, M.; Pan, C.; et al. Fusobacterium nucleatum Increases Proliferation of Colorectal Cancer Cells and Tumor Development in Mice by Activating Toll-Like Receptor 4 Signaling to Nuclear Factor-κB, and Up-regulating Expression of MicroRNA-21. *Gastroenterology* **2017**, *152*, 851–866.e24. [CrossRef] [PubMed]
45. Baroni, A.; Orlando, M.; Donnarumma, G.; Farro, P.; Iovene, M.R.; Tufano, M.A.; Buommino, E. Toll-like receptor 2 (TLR2) mediates intracellular signalling in human keratinocytes in response to Malassezia furfur. *Arch. Dermatol. Res.* **2006**, *297*, 280–288. [CrossRef]
46. Burrows, M.P.; Volchkov, P.; Kobayashi, K.S.; Chervonsky, A.V. Microbiota regulates type 1 diabetes through Toll-like receptors. *Proc. Natl. Acad. Sci. USA* **2015**, *112*, 9973–9977. [CrossRef]

47. Singer-Englar, T.; Barlow, G.; Mathur, R. Obesity, diabetes, and the gut microbiome: An updated review. *Expert. Rev. Gastroenterol. Hepatol.* **2019**, *13*, 3–15. [CrossRef]
48. Simon, M.C.; Reinbeck, A.L.; Wessel, C.; Heindirk, J.; Jelenik, T.; Kaul, K.; Arreguin-Cano, J.; Strom, A.; Blaut, M.; Bäckhed, F.; et al. Distinct alterations of gut morphology and microbiota characterize accelerated diabetes onset in nonobese diabetic mice. *J. Biol. Chem.* **2020**, *295*, 969–980. [CrossRef]

Disclaimer/Publisher's Note: The statements, opinions and data contained in all publications are solely those of the individual author(s) and contributor(s) and not of MDPI and/or the editor(s). MDPI and/or the editor(s) disclaim responsibility for any injury to people or property resulting from any ideas, methods, instructions or products referred to in the content.

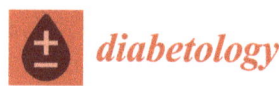 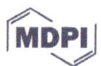

Commentary

Sodium-Glucose Co-Transporter 2 Inhibitors as a Powerful Cardioprotective and Renoprotective Tool: Overview of Clinical Trials and Mechanisms

Andrej Belančić [1,2,*] and Sanja Klobučar [3,4]

1. Department of Clinical Pharmacology, Clinical Hospital Centre Rijeka, 51000 Rijeka, Croatia
2. Department of Basic and Clinical Pharmacology with Toxicology, Faculty of Medicine, University of Rijeka, 51000 Rijeka, Croatia
3. Department of Internal Medicine, Division of Endocrinology, Diabetes and Metabolic Diseases, Clinical Hospital Centre Rijeka, 51000 Rijeka, Croatia; sanja.klobucarm@gmail.com
4. Department of Internal Medicine, Faculty of Medicine, University of Rijeka, 51000 Rijeka, Croatia
* Correspondence: a.belancic93@gmail.com or andrej.belancic@uniri.hr

Abstract: Sodium-glucose co-transporter 2 (SGLT2) inhibitors have been linked to beneficial effects on cardiovascular risk factors, blood pressure, body weight, and lipid profile, according to a substantial body of literature. Significant cardiac and renal benefits with the use of SGLT2 inhibitors have been shown in patients with type 2 diabetes, as well as in those with heart failure and/or chronic kidney disease (CKD), regardless of diabetes status, in subsequent large cardiovascular outcome trials. Thus, SGLT2 inhibitors have become a mainstay of therapy for type 2 diabetes in patients with established cardiovascular disease and CKD due to their benefits for the heart and kidneys. Based on data from randomized controlled trials and meta-analyses, this article attempts to present a thorough review of the mechanism of action, as well as the benefits of SGLT2 inhibitors for cardiac and renal protection. On the basis of a growing body of literature on diabetes and other conditions, clinical practice guidelines have been updated to suggest the use of SGLT2 inhibitors in specific patient populations. These modifications will also be concisely described, based on evidence-based medicine principles.

Keywords: antidiabetic; antihyperglycemic; cardioprotection; cardiovascular outcome trial; clinical trials; diabetes; pharmacology; renal outcomes; renoprotection; sodium-glucose co-transporter 2 inhibitors

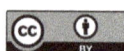

1. Introduction

Sodium-glucose co-transporter 2 inhibitors (SGLT2i) are the latest class of antihyperglycemic drugs for the treatment of type 2 diabetes mellitus. Four SGLT2 inhibitors (dapagliflozin, empagliflozin, canagliflozin, and ertugliflozin) are currently authorized in the European Union and are available on the market as monocomponent drugs or in combination with metformin or dipeptidyl peptidase 4 inhibitors [1,2]. SGLT2 inhibition reduces glucose reabsorption from glomerular filtrate in the proximal renal tubule and at the same time sodium reabsorption, ultimately achieving glycosuria (and consequently, regulation of fasting and postprandial glycemia), natriuresis, and osmotic diuresis. It should be noted that the amount of glucose that the kidney eliminates by this glucose mechanism is dependent on the concentration of glucose in the blood and on the rate of glomerular filtration (GFR). Furthermore, increased delivery of sodium to the distal tubule increases tubuloglomerular feedback and reduces intraglomerular pressure, which in combination with osmotic diuresis consequently leads to a decrease in preload and afterload, and thus, among other things, has beneficial effects on cardiac remodeling and preservation of renal function [2–4].

SGLT2i has shown good efficacy and tolerability in the treatment of people with type 2 diabetes mellitus, regardless of the duration of the disease and the function of β-cells of Langerhans islets. According to meta-analyses of clinical studies, the use of SGLT2 inhibitors achieves a noticeable effect on the regulation of fasting and postprandial glycemia, with an average decrease in glycated haemoglobin (HbA1c) of about 0.5–1%, without increasing the risk of hypoglycemia. This group of drugs generally has a good safety profile, and the most common side effects (urinary tract infections, vulvovaginal candidiasis, polyuria, polakysuria) are precisely the product of the basic pharmacological glycosuric effect. A rare but serious adverse reaction that may occur during treatment with SGLT2 inhibitors is (euglycemic) ketoacidosis, the mechanism of which has not yet been fully understood, but it is known to occur more frequently in type 1 diabetes mellitus patients (which is why dapagliflozin recently abolished the indication for type 1 diabetes mellitus). According to meta-analytic data, no significant differences in safety profile between different SGLT2 inhibitor agents were shown generally [5]. Other beneficial effects of SGLT2 inhibition, in addition to the basic glycemic effects, are cardioprotection, renoprotection, and antiobesogenic effect (loss of energy/calories and reduction in body weight $\approx$ 2 kg) [6–9].

Based on data from randomized controlled trials and meta-analyses, this article attempts to present a thorough review of the mechanism of action, as well as the benefits of SGLT2 inhibitors for cardiac and renal protection. Clinical practice guidelines have been updated to suggest the use of SGLT2 inhibitors in specific patient populations regardless of diabetes status. Thus, these modifications will also be concisely described, based on evidence-based medicine principles.

2. Cardiovascular and Renal Events in the Setting of Type 2 Diabetes Mellitus Clinical Trials

Encouraged by the adverse cardiovascular effects of rosiglitazone, the Food and Drug Administration (FDA) since 2008 and the European Medicines Agency (EMA) since 2012, in addition to the standard evidence of antihyperglycemic efficacy and safety, require evidence from randomized double-blind placebo-controlled clinical studies on the effect of the antihyperglycemic agent on cardiovascular outcomes (CV Outcome Trial; CVOT). The primary outcome measure of the latter studies is the time until the first occurrence of a major adverse cardiovascular event (MACE, which is a composite of death due to cardiovascular cause, myocardial infarction, or ischemic stroke) [10]. To highlight, valid conclusions can be drawn from studies solely on the basis of primary outcomes (e.g., MACE here), while this should not be done on the basis of secondary outcomes (which are exclusively affirmative) due to insufficient statistical strength. In addition to the primary MACE outcomes, this paragraph will also present isolated secondary renal outcomes and outcomes for heart failure (HF) of some conducted CVOTs purely because they have hinted towards the renoprotective effects of SGLT2i and beneficial effects on chronic heart failure and thus set the need to conduct further targeted trials primarily designed to demonstrate the effectiveness of some representatives in these indications [11–13].

The EMPA-REG OUTCOME study (n = 7020; median follow-up of 3.1 years) demonstrated a 14% relative reduction in MACE in subjects receiving empagliflozin (HR (hazard ratio) 0.86, 95% CI (confidence interval) 0.74–0.99; p = 0.04 for superiority). Empagliflozin reduced the risk of heart failure that would require hospitalization compared to placebo (2.7% vs. 4.1%, HR 0.65, 95% CI 0.50–0.85; p = 0.002; the secondary outcome). Furthermore, the investigational drug hinted towards possible beneficial effects in terms of slowing down the rate of eGFR reduction, given the results obtained in terms of secondary MARE outcomes (doubling of serum creatinine levels with eGFR $\leq$ 45, initiation of renal function replacement or death due to renal cause)—HR 0.54, 95% CI 0.40–0.75, $p \leq$ 0.001 [14]. Canagliflozin demonstrated superiority (HR 0.86, 95% CI 0.75–0.97, p = 0.02 for superiority) over placebo in the MACE reduction in the CANVAS study (n = 10,142, median follow-up of 2.4 years). In terms of secondary outcomes, the group of subjects who received canagliflozin had a significantly lower risk of heart failure that would require hospitalization (HR 0.67, 95% CI 0.52–0.87), and some renal benefit was already suggested [15]. The latter was later confirmed in CREDENCE, a double-blind, randomized, placebo-controlled study, involving patients with an eGFR of 30–90 and albuminuria (albumin/creatinine 300–5000 mg/g) who had concomitant medicamentous blockade of the renin–angiotensin system. The primary outcome was composite, and it consisted of the terminal stage of CKD (dialysis, kidney transplantation, eGFR < 15), doubling the values of serum creatinine, or death due to renal or cardiovascular cause. The study was completed earlier (median follow-up 2.6 years; 4401 subjects randomized), since the planned interim analysis verified a 30% relative reduction in this MARCE composite outcome (HR 0.70, 95% CI 0.59–0.82, $p = 0.00001$) [16]. Furthermore, in the DECLARE-TIMI 58 study (n = 17,160, median follow-up for 4.2 years), a non-inferiority of dapagliflozin to placebo in terms of MACE reduction (HR 0.93, 95% CI 0.84–1.03), as well as superiority in terms of co-primary composite outcome resulting from cardiovascular death or hospitalization for heart failure (4.9% vs. 5.8%, HR 0.83, 95% CI 0.73–0.95; $p = 0.005$; primarily at the expense of heart failure outcome HR 0.73, 95% CI 0.61–0.88) were detected. Among the secondary outcomes of this study was MARCE composite outcome (40% reduction in eGFR with its value < 60, progression to the terminal stage of CKD including the need for renal function replacement, or death due to renal or cardiovascular cause, where its 47% relative reduction was achieved along with dapagliflozin (HR 0.53, 95% CI 0.43–0.66, $p < 0.001$) [17]. Finally, ertugliflozin in the VERTIS CV study (n = 8246, median follow-up of 3.5 years) proved to be exclusively non-inferior to placebo in terms of MACE reduction (HR 0.97, 95% CI 0.85–1.11, $p < 0.001$ for non-inferiority). Among secondary outcomes, HR for hospitalization for heart failure was 0.70 (95% CI 0.54–0.90), while for MARE it was 0.81 (95% CI 0.63–1.04) [18].

Given the surprisingly favorable cardiovascular and renal benefits of individual SGLT2i representatives, further targeted clinical trials on the effectiveness of SGLT2 inhibition in chronic heart failure and chronic kidney disease (CKD) were conducted. Thus, in recent years, we are able to prescribe dapagliflozin for the treatment of HF with reduced ejection fraction (HFrEF) and CKD and empagliflozin for the treatment of HFrEF, HF with mildly reduced EF (HFmrEF), and HF with preserved EF (HFpEF), both regardless of the existence of type 2 diabetes mellitus.

3. Cardioprotective Effects and Mechanisms of SGLT2 Inhibitors

Cardioprotective effects of SGLT2 inhibition are associated with (i) reduction in preload (natriuresis, osmotic diuresis) and afterload (reduction in blood pressure, improvement of vascular function), which consequently carries favorable effects on cardiac remodeling, (ii) improvement of cardiac metabolism and bioenergetics, (iii) inhibition of myocardial Na+/H+ exchange, (iv) reduction in cardiac fibrosis and necrosis, and (v) alteration of the production of adipokines, cytokines, and the amount of epicardial adipose tissue. Certainly, in addition to the above, the overall cardioprotection is indirectly (secondarily) contributed by the associated antiobesogenic effect, reduction in blood pressure, reduction in stiffness of the arteries, as well as better regulation of glycemia [19–21].

Dapagliflozin demonstrated efficacy and safety in the treatment of HFrEF (≤40%) in the DAPA-HF clinical study. It was a double-blind randomized placebo-controlled clinical study that involved 4744 patients with HFrEF (≤40%) and NYHA (New York Heart Association) stage II–IV, with or without diabetes. After 1.5 years of follow-up, a 26% relative reduction with dapagliflozin at a dose of 10 mg per os/day was achieved in terms of primary composite outcome (death from cardiovascular cause or worsening of heart failure—hospitalization for heart failure or visit to the emergency tract due to the need for parenteral diuretic therapy)—HF 0.74, 95% CI 0.65–0.85, $p < 0.001$. The latter benefit was demonstrated in both patients with (n = 2139) and without (n = 2605) diabetes mellitus, and the safety profile was congruent with that previously known from clinical studies with dapagliflozin for type 2 diabetes [22]. Furthermore, the EMPEROR-Reduced clinical study proved the efficacy and safety of empagliflozin (10 mg/day per os) in the treatment of HFrEF. There were 3730 randomized subjects (1:1) who were followed for 1.3 years; subjects receiving empagliflozin had a 25% relative reduction in primary composite outcome (death from cardiovascular cause or hospitalization due to heart failure)—HR 0.75, 95% CI 0.65–0.86, $p < 0.001$. The analysis of the subgroups again proved that this benefit is evident in both subjects with (n = 1856) and without (n = 1874) diabetes mellitus [23]. Consequently, the SGLT-2 inhibitor (empagliflozin or dapagliflozin at a dose of 10 mg per os/day) was included in the recent guidelines of the European Society of Cardiology for the treatment of HFrEF with the aim of reducing the risk of hospitalization and cardiovascular mortality—recommendation Ia [24].

In the double-blind placebo-controlled EMPEROR-Preserved study (n = 5988, median follow-up of 26.2 months), empagliflozin also showed potential in the treatment of HF with ejection fraction >40%. It achieved a 21% relative reduction in terms of primary composite outcome consisting of death from cardiovascular cause or hospitalization for heart failure—HR 0.79, 95% CI 0.69–0.90, $p < 0.001$, and mostly at the expense of reducing the risk of hospitalization due to heart failure (27% relative reduction) [25]. It should be noted that further clinical studies (e.g., DELIVER study) are still being conducted to assess the effectiveness of SGLT2 inhibition in HF with a medium range of ejection fraction (mrEF; 41–49%) and with preserved ejection fraction (pEF; $\geq$50%), in order to achieve an even stronger body of evidence for SGLT2i prescription in this indication. For instance, in the DELIVER study (n = 6264), dapagliflozin reduced the combined risk of worsening heart failure or cardiovascular death among patients with heart failure and a mildly reduced or preserved ejection fraction by 18%—HR 0.82, 95% CI 0.73–0.92, $p < 0.001$ [26].

Finally, according to recent relevant meta-analytic data, SGLT2i reduced the risk of cardiovascular death and hospitalizations for HF in a broad range of patients with HF, irrespective of ejection fraction or care setting [27].

Last but not least, it would be useful in further randomized clinical studies to separately evaluate the effectiveness of SGLT2 inhibition in patients with medium range and those with preserved ejection fraction, given the different pathophysiological bases and clinical determinants HFmrEF and HFpEF.

4. Renoprotective Effects and Mechanisms of SGLT2 Inhibitors

The mechanism of renoprotection of SGLT2 inhibitors has not yet been fully understood. However, one of the most important renoprotective mechanisms is the restoration of tubuloglomerular feedback by increasing the delivery of sodium to the distal tubule (macula densa), i.e., the consequent constriction of the afferent arteriole and the reduction in glomerular hyperfiltration. The second proposed mechanism is actually related to the latter because it is a decrease in the degree of activity of the renal renin–angiotensin–aldosterone system, which also contributes to the reduction in glomerular hyperfiltration, i.e., intraglomerular pressure. Other possible secondary mechanisms mentioned in the literature are (i) a slightly more pronounced production of ketone bodies (β-hydroxy butyrate), which are then used as an alternative fuel for the production of adenosine triphosphate in mitochondria and thus help the attenuation of inflammation, and (ii) the effect of protection against hypoxia, oxidative stress, and fibrosis (extensively presented elsewhere [28,29]).

In the DAPA-CKD study, 4304 subjects with chronic kidney disease (eGFR 25–75 and albuminuria—albumin/creatinine ratio of 200–5000 mg/g) were randomized to receive dapagliflozin at a dose of 10 mg or placebo, on top of concomitant medicamentous blockade of the renin–angiotensin system. The median follow-up was 2.4 years, and the primary MARCE composite outcome of the study included a sustained reduction in eGFR by $\geq$50%, end-stage renal disease (chronic dialysis, kidney transplantation, eGFR < 15), or death due to cardiovascular or renal cause. Subjects receiving dapagliflozin achieved a 39% relative reduction in terms of primary MARCE outcome (HR 0.61, 95% CI 0.51–0.72, $p < 0.001$). All four components of the primary unified outcome measure individually contributed to this therapeutic effect, and the benefit was present in patients with and without diabetes [30]. In the randomized, double-blind, placebo-controlled EMPA-KIDNEY trial, patients' responses to empagliflozin were assessed in two groups: those with GFRs of 20 to 45 and any albumin-to-creatinine ratio, and those with GFRs of 45 to 90 and at least

200 ACR. The study randomized 6609 patients to either empagliflozin 10 mg once daily or placebo. When compared to the placebo group, those who were taking empagliflozin had significantly lower rates of CKD development and mortality from CV causes at the 2-year median follow-up (13.1% vs. 16.9%, respectively; HR 0.72 [0.64 to 0.82], $p = 0.001$). These findings persisted across all CKD levels and among patients with and without diabetes [31].

Finally, recent meta-analytic data of randomized controlled trials support their use for modifying risk of kidney disease progression and acute kidney injury, not only in patients with type 2 diabetes at high cardiovascular risk, but also in patients with chronic kidney disease or heart failure irrespective of diabetes status, primary kidney disease, or kidney function [32].

5. Brief Discussion on Existing Challenges and Gaps in the Research and Application of SGLT2 Inhibitors

Despite the undeniable cardiorenal clinical benefit of SGLT2i, a notable percentage of non-diabetic patients with HF or CKD still do not receive these medications. Some physicians still reference them exclusively as antihyperglycemic or "diabetes" drugs. The latter may be due to various barriers and limitations such as clinical inertia, lack of familiarity of physicians with the evidence-based practice and current guidelines, non-promotion of cross-disciplinarity, cost, availability, etc. [33,34]

It would be important to directly identify and investigate the relative importance of each factor in prescribing practices. A collaborative multidisciplinary effort at the local, national, and international levels should be undertaken to address and resolve clinical inertia by doing the following: (i) identifying barriers and practices to change; (ii) improving knowledge of how to weigh risks and benefits on a case-by-case basis (phenotype principle); (iii) advocating for post-CVOT treatment pathways; (iv) advocating for local guidelines and collaborating on local educational initiatives; (v) fostering interdisciplinary collaboration; (vi) educating and updating reimbursement authorities on new clinical data; (vi) helping patients understand the benefits and goals of cardiorenal protection; and (vii) measuring the performance of individual clinicians to provide feedback and incentivize change [35].

It is of interest to understand which patients (phenotype influence) benefit most from the cardiorenal protection provided by SGLT2 inhibitor therapy, independent of diabetes status or glycemic control.

Another issue that future research should address is the question of (non)discontinuation of SGLT2i after the episode of euglycemic diabetic ketoacidosis on a case-by-case basis, taking into account the recent evidence on mortality reduction, cardiac and renal protection, etc. [36]

In addition, continued patient monitoring (both for effectiveness and safety profile) and longer-term real-world clinical data collection on SGLT2 inhibition in different comorbidities, as well as head-to-head comparisons between different SGLT2 inhibitors and with different treatment modalities of proven benefit, are extremely important [37]. This is even more important from the perspective of patient groups that are generally underrepresented in clinical trials (e.g., older adults) and for whom relevant secondary outcomes (e.g., functional status and quality of life) were not included in the study design [38].

To evaluate the effects of SGLT2i drugs on glomerular disorders, reduced eGFR, non-proteinuric CKD, dialysis and transplant populations, HFmrEF and HFpEF, and other diseases, the results of upcoming studies are eagerly awaited.

6. Conclusions

SGLT2 inhibitors, in addition to their already known antihyperglycemic and antiobesogenic effects, have been shown to be beneficial in terms of cardioprotection, renal protection, and thus, more recently, as a valuable form of therapy in chronic heart failure and chronic kidney disease, regardless of the presence of diabetes. Thus, SGLT2 inhibitors are becoming an increasingly valued medical resource in the field of endocrinology, cardiology, and nephrology. For this reason, it is very important to improve the knowledge of physicians of all specialties about this promising group of drugs so that they can be better integrated into clinical practice in all indications for which they have shown indisputable benefits in randomized clinical trials.

Author Contributions: A.B. and S.K. contributed equally to this work. Both authors were involved in writing the paper and had final approval of the submitted version. All authors have read and agreed to the published version of the manuscript.

Funding: This research received no external funding.

Institutional Review Board Statement: Not applicable.

Informed Consent Statement: Not applicable.

Data Availability Statement: Not applicable.

Conflicts of Interest: A.B. declares no conflict of interest. S.K. has served as principal investigator or co-investigator in clinical trials of Eli Lilly, MSD, Novo Nordisk, and Sanofi Aventis. She has received honoraria for speaking or advisory board engagements and consulting fees from Abbott, AstraZeneca, Boehringer Ingelheim, Eli Lilly, Novartis, Novo Nordisk, MSD, Mylan, Sanofi Aventis, and Servier.

Abbreviations

CI	confidence interval
CKD	chronic kidney disease
CVOT	cardiovascular outcomes trial
GFR	glomerular filtration
HbA1c	glycated hemoglobin
HF	heart failure
HR	hazard ratio
mrEF	mildly reduced ejection fraction
NYHA	New York Hear Association
pEF	preserved ejection fraction
rEF	reduced ejection fraction
SGLT2i	Sodium-glucose co-transporter 2 inhibitors

References

1. Rahelić, D.; Altabas, V.; Bakula, M.; Balić, S.; Balint, I.; Marković, B.B.; Bicanić, N.; Bjelinski, I.; Bozikov, V.; Varzić, S.C.; et al. Croatian guidelines for the pharmacotherapy of type 2 diabetes. *Lijec. Vjesn.* **2016**, *138*, 1–21.
2. European Medicines Agency. Available online: https://www.ema.europa.eu/en/medicines (accessed on 12 June 2023).
3. Scheen, A.J. Pharmacodynamics, efficacy and safety of sodium-glucose co-transporter type 2 (SGLT2) inhibitors for the treatment of type 2 diabetes mellitus. *Drugs* **2015**, *75*, 33–59. [CrossRef]
4. Wright, E.M. SGLT2 Inhibitors: Physiology and Pharmacology. *Kidney360* **2021**, *17*, 2027–2037. [CrossRef]
5. Donnan, J.R.; Grandy, C.A.; Chibrikov, E.; Marra, C.A.; Aubrey-Bassler, K.; Johnston, K.; Swab, M.; Hache, J.; Curnew, D.; Nguyen, H.; et al. Comparative safety of the sodium glucose co-transporter 2 (SGLT2) inhibitors: A systematic review and meta-analysis. *BMJ Open* **2019**, *9*, e022577. [CrossRef] [PubMed]
6. Musso, G.; Gambino, R.; Cassader, M.; Pagano, G. A novel approach to control hyperglycemia in type 2 diabetes: Sodium glucose co-transport (SGLT) inhibitors: Systematic review and meta-analysis of randomized trials. *Ann. Med.* **2012**, *44*, 375–393. [CrossRef]
7. Clar, C.; Gill, J.A.; Court, R.; Waugh, N. Systematic review of SGLT2 receptor inhibitors in dual or triple therapy in type 2 diabetes. *BMJ Open* **2012**, *2*, e001007. [CrossRef]
8. Vasilakou, D.; Karagiannis, T.; Athanasiadou, E.; Mainou, M.; Liakos, A.; Bekiari, E.; Sarigianni, M.; Matthews, D.R.; Tsapas, A. Sodium-glucose cotransporter 2 inhibitors for type 2 diabetes: A systematic review and meta-analysis. *Ann. Intern. Med.* **2013**, *159*, 262–274. [CrossRef] [PubMed]
9. Berhan, A.; Barker, A. Sodium glucose co-transport 2 inhibitors in the treatment of type 2 diabetes mellitus: A meta-analysis of randomized double-blind controlled trials. *BMC Endocr. Disord.* **2013**, *13*, 58. [CrossRef]
10. Lo, C.W.H.; Fei, Y.; Cheung, B.M.Y. Cardiovascular Outcomes in Trials of New Antidiabetic Drug Classes. *Card. Fail. Rev.* **2021**, *7*, e04. [CrossRef]
11. Mazin, I.; Chernomordik, F.; Fefer, P.; Matetzky, S.; Beigel, R. The Impact of Novel Anti-Diabetic Medications on CV Outcomes: A New Therapeutic Horizon for Diabetic and Non-Diabetic Cardiac Patients. *J. Clin. Med.* **2022**, *11*, 1904. [CrossRef] [PubMed]

12. Rangaswami, J.; Bhalla, V.; de Boer, I.H.; Staruschenko, A.; Sharp, J.A.; Singh, R.R.; Lo, K.B.; Tuttle, K.; Vaduganathan, M.; Ventura, H.; et al. Cardiorenal Protection With the Newer Antidiabetic Agents in Patients With Diabetes and Chronic Kidney Disease: A Scientific Statement From the American Heart Association. *Circulation* **2020**, *142*, e265–e286. [CrossRef]
13. Ferro, E.G.; Elshazly, M.B.; Bhatt, D.L. New Antidiabetes Medications and Their Cardiovascular and Renal Benefits. *Cardiol. Clin.* **2021**, *39*, 335–351. [CrossRef]
14. Zinman, B.; Wanner, C.; Lachin, J.M.; Fitchett, D.; Bluhmki, E.; Hantel, S.; Mattheus, M.; Devins, T.; Johansen, O.E.; Woerle, H.J.; et al. Empagliflozin, Cardiovascular Outcomes, and Mortality in Type 2 Diabetes. *N. Engl. J. Med.* **2015**, *373*, 2117–2128. [CrossRef]
15. Khokhlov, A.; Vorobjev, S.; Mirolyubova, O.; Boldueva, S.; Ershova, O.; Ballyzek, M.; Smolenskaya, O.; Yakushin, S.S.; Zateyshchikov, D.; Arkhipov, M.; et al. Canagliflozin and Cardiovascular and Renal Events in Type 2 Diabetes. *N. Engl. J. Med.* **2017**, *377*, 644–657. [CrossRef]
16. Perkovic, V.; Jardine, M.J.; Neal, B.; Bompoint, S.; Heerspink, H.J.L.; Charytan, D.M.; Edwards, R.; Agarwal, R.; Bakris, G.; Bull, S.; et al. Canagliflozin and Renal Outcomes in Type 2 Diabetes and Nephropathy. *N. Engl. J. Med.* **2019**, *380*, 2295–2306. [CrossRef] [PubMed]
17. Wiviott, S.D.; Raz, I.; Bonaca, M.P.; Mosenzon, O.; Kato, E.T.; Cahn, A.; Silverman, M.G.; Zelniker, T.A.; Kuder, J.F.; Murphy, S.A.; et al. Dapagliflozin and Cardiovascular Outcomes in Type 2 Diabetes. *N. Engl. J. Med.* **2019**, *380*, 347–357. [CrossRef]
18. Cannon, C.P.; Pratley, R.; Dagogo-Jack, S.; Mancuso, J.; Huyck, S.; Masiukiewicz, U.; Charbonnel, B.; Frederich, R.; Gallo, S.; Cosentino, F.; et al. Cardiovascular Outcomes with Ertugliflozin in Type 2 Diabetes. *N. Engl. J. Med.* **2020**, *383*, 1425–1435. [CrossRef]
19. Verma, S.; McMurray, J.J.V. SGLT2 inhibitors and mechanisms of cardiovascular benefit: A state-of-the-art review. *Diabetologia* **2018**, *61*, 2108–2117. [CrossRef] [PubMed]
20. Lopaschuk, G.D.; Verma, S. Mechanisms of Cardiovascular Benefits of Sodium Glucose Co-Transporter 2 (SGLT2) Inhibitors: A State-of-the-Art Review. *JACC Basic Transl. Sci.* **2020**, *5*, 632–644. [CrossRef]
21. Salvatore, T.; Galiero, R.; Caturano, A.; Rinaldi, L.; Di Martino, A.; Albanese, G.; Di Salvo, J.; Epifani, R.; Marfella, R.; Docimo, G.; et al. An Overview of the Cardiorenal Protective Mechanisms of SGLT2 Inhibitors. *Int. J. Mol. Sci.* **2022**, *23*, 3651. [CrossRef]
22. McMurray, J.J.V.; Solomon, S.D.; Inzucchi, S.E.; Køber, L.; Kosiborod, M.N.; Martinez, F.A.; Ponikowski, P.; Sabatine, M.S.; Anand, I.S.; Bělohlávek, J.; et al. Dapagliflozin in Patients with Heart Failure and Reduced Ejection Fraction. *N. Engl. J. Med.* **2019**, *381*, 1995–2008. [CrossRef] [PubMed]
23. Packer, M.; Anker, S.D.; Butler, J.; Filippatos, G.; Pocock, S.J.; Carson, P.; Januzzi, J.; Verma, S.; Tsutsui, H.; Brueckmann, M.; et al. Cardiovascular and Renal Outcomes with Empagliflozin in Heart Failure. *N. Engl. J. Med.* **2020**, *383*, 1413–1424. [CrossRef] [PubMed]
24. McDonagh, T.A.; Metra, M.; Adamo, M.; Gardner, R.S.; Baumbach, A.; Böhm, M.; Burri, H.; Butler, J.; Čelutkienė, J.; Chioncel, O.; et al. 2021 ESC Guidelines for the diagnosis and treatment of acute and chronic heart failure: Developed by the Task Force for the diagnosis and treatment of acute and chronic heart failure of the European Society of Cardiology (ESC). With the special contribution of the Heart Failure Association (HFA) of the ESC. *Eur. J. Heart Fail.* **2022**, *24*, 4–131. [CrossRef]
25. Anker, S.D.; Butler, J.; Filippatos, G.; Ferreira, J.P.; Bocchi, E.; Böhm, M.; Brunner-La Rocca, H.P.; Choi, D.J.; Chopra, V.; Chuquiure-Valenzuela, E.; et al. Empagliflozin in Heart Failure with a Preserved Ejection Fraction. *N. Engl. J. Med.* **2021**, *385*, 1451–1461. [CrossRef]
26. Solomon, S.D.; McMurray, J.J.V.; Claggett, B.; de Boer, R.A.; DeMets, D.; Hernandez, A.F.; Inzucchi, S.E.; Kosiborod, M.N.; Lam, C.S.P.; Martinez, F.; et al. Dapagliflozin in Heart Failure with Mildly Reduced or Preserved Ejection Fraction. *N. Engl. J. Med.* **2022**, *387*, 1089–1098. [CrossRef]
27. Vaduganathan, M.; Docherty, K.F.; Claggett, B.L.; Jhund, P.S.; de Boer, R.A.; Hernandez, A.F.; Inzucchi, S.E.; Kosiborod, M.N.; Lam, C.S.P.; Martinez, F.; et al. SGLT-2 inhibitors in patients with heart failure: A comprehensive meta-analysis of five randomised controlled trials. *Lancet* **2022**, *400*, 757–767. [CrossRef]
28. Ravindran, S.; Munusamy, S. Renoprotective mechanisms of sodium-glucose co-transporter 2 (SGLT2) inhibitors against the progression of diabetic kidney disease. *J. Cell Physiol.* **2022**, *237*, 1182–1205. [CrossRef]
29. Skrabic, R.; Kumric, M.; Vrdoljak, J.; Rusic, D.; Skrabic, I.; Vilovic, M.; Martinovic, D.; Duplancic, V.; Ticinovic Kurir, T.; Bozic, J. SGLT2 Inhibitors in Chronic Kidney Disease: From Mechanisms to Clinical Practice. *Biomedicines* **2022**, *10*, 2458. [CrossRef] [PubMed]
30. Heerspink, H.J.L.; Stefánsson, B.V.; Correa-Rotter, R.; Chertow, G.M.; Greene, T.; Hou, F.F.; Mann, J.F.E.; McMurray, J.J.V.; Lindberg, M.; Rossing, P.; et al. Dapagliflozin in Patients with Chronic Kidney Disease. *N. Engl. J. Med.* **2020**, *383*, 1436–1446. [CrossRef]
31. Herrington, W.G.; Staplin, N.; Wanner, C.; Green, J.B.; Hauske, S.J.; Emberson, J.R.; Preiss, D.; Judge, P.; Mayne, K.J.; Ng, S.Y.A.; et al. Empagliflozin in Patients with Chronic Kidney Disease. *N. Engl. J. Med.* **2023**, *388*, 117–127. [CrossRef]
32. Nuffield Department of Population Health Renal Studies Group; SGLT2 inhibitor Meta-Analysis Cardio-Renal Trialists' Consortium. Impact of diabetes on the effects of sodium glucose co-transporter-2 inhibitors on kidney outcomes: Collaborative meta-analysis of large placebo-controlled trials. *Lancet* **2022**, *400*, 1788–1801. [CrossRef] [PubMed]
33. Adhikari, R.; Jha, K.; Dardari, Z.; Heyward, J.; Blumenthal, R.S.; Eckel, R.H.; Alexander, G.C.; Blaha, M.J. National Trends in Use of Sodium-Glucose Cotransporter-2 Inhibitors and Glucagon-like Peptide-1 Receptor Agonists by Cardiologists and Other Specialties, 2015 to 2020. *J. Am. Heart Assoc.* **2022**, *11*, e023811. [CrossRef] [PubMed]

34. Krishnan, A.; Shankar, M.; Lerma, E.V.; Wiegley, N.; GlomCon Editorial Team. Sodium Glucose Cotransporter 2 (SGLT2) Inhibitors and CKD: Are You a #Flozinator? *Kidney Med.* **2023**, *5*, 100608. [CrossRef] [PubMed]
35. Schernthaner, G.; Shehadeh, N.; Ametov, A.S.; Bazarova, A.V.; Ebrahimi, F.; Fasching, P.; Janež, A.; Kempler, P.; Konrāde, I.; Lalić, N.M.; et al. Worldwide inertia to the use of cardiorenal protective glucose-lowering drugs (SGLT2i and GLP-1 RA) in high-risk patients with type 2 diabetes. *Cardiovasc. Diabetol.* **2020**, *19*, 185. [CrossRef]
36. Selwyn, J.; Pichardo-Lowden, A.R. Managing Hospitalized Patients Taking SGLT2 Inhibitors: Reducing the Risk of Euglycemic Diabetic Ketoacidosis. *Diabetology* **2023**, *4*, 86–92. [CrossRef]
37. Fadini, G.P.; Del Prato, S.; Avogaro, A.; Solini, A. Challenges and opportunities in real-world evidence on the renal effects of sodium-glucose cotransporter-2 inhibitors. *Diabetes Obes. Metab.* **2022**, *24*, 177–186. [CrossRef]
38. Bellary, S.; Barnett, A.H. SGLT2 inhibitors in older adults: Overcoming the age barrier. *Lancet Healthy Longev.* **2023**, *4*, e127–e128. [CrossRef]

Disclaimer/Publisher's Note: The statements, opinions and data contained in all publications are solely those of the individual author(s) and contributor(s) and not of MDPI and/or the editor(s). MDPI and/or the editor(s) disclaim responsibility for any injury to people or property resulting from any ideas, methods, instructions or products referred to in the content.

MDPI AG
Grosspeteranlage 5
4052 Basel
Switzerland
Tel.: +41 61 683 77 34

Diabetology Editorial Office
E-mail: diabetology@mdpi.com
www.mdpi.com/journal/diabetology

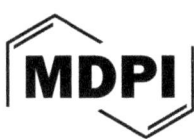

Disclaimer/Publisher's Note: The statements, opinions and data contained in all publications are solely those of the individual author(s) and contributor(s) and not of MDPI and/or the editor(s). MDPI and/or the editor(s) disclaim responsibility for any injury to people or property resulting from any ideas, methods, instructions or products referred to in the content.